The Joy of Pregnancy

The Joy of Pregnancy

Mary Brandt Kerr

MEDICAL CONSULTANT

J. MERVYN LLOYD M.D.

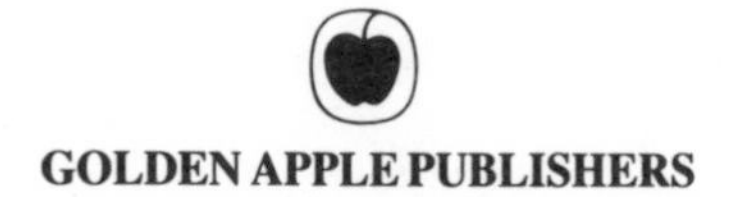

GOLDEN APPLE PUBLISHERS

The information and recommendations contained in this book are intended to complement, not substitute for, the advice of your own physician. Before starting any medical treatment, exercise program or diet, consult your physician. Information in this book is given without any guarantees on the part of the author, Footnote Productions Limited, The Quarto Group Inc. or Golden Apple Publishers and they cannot be held responsible for the contents in this book.

The Joy of Pregnancy

A Golden Apple Publication
Published by arrangement with
Footnote Productions Limited
A Division of the Quarto Group, Inc.

June 1987

Printed in Hong Kong

987654321

ISBN 0-553-19917-X

CONTENTS

YOU'RE PREGNANT? CONGRATULATIONS!

The news that you're pregnant can be the most joyous you'll ever receive. It means you're about to enter a nine-month period of tremendous change and growth—both for you and your partner. And at the end of it, you'll embark on a lifelong voyage as a parent, with all the special joys that brings as you watch your child grow.

The news that you're pregnant also brings a flood of emotions. The chief feeling is utter delight, mixed with a lot of eager anticipation. But you may also feel a little frightened and have a lot of questions. The more you know about what to expect as your baby develops, the more confident you will feel, and the more you can enjoy your pregnancy. This book will answer many of your questions, but you are sure to have many more. Never hesitate to ask your doctor or midwife *any* question you may have—he or she will be only too happy to answer. After all, the more secure and happy you are about your pregnancy, the better for everyone.

As your pregnancy advances, you will have to cope with your changing body and your changing emotions. It's a time that requires a lot of understanding from your partner, but don't forget that he too is experiencing a lot of emotional change. Be open with each other, be patient, and remember that your love for each other has led you to create a baby *together*.

Pregnancy is not only a time of great physical change, *but also of introspection. The emotions of delight, anxiety, anticipation and worry over your new parental responsibilities may follow each other with bewildering speed. Careful reading and preparation for the birth will help allay fears and keep you in touch with what is happening to your body, leaving you free to enjoy the coming months to the full.*

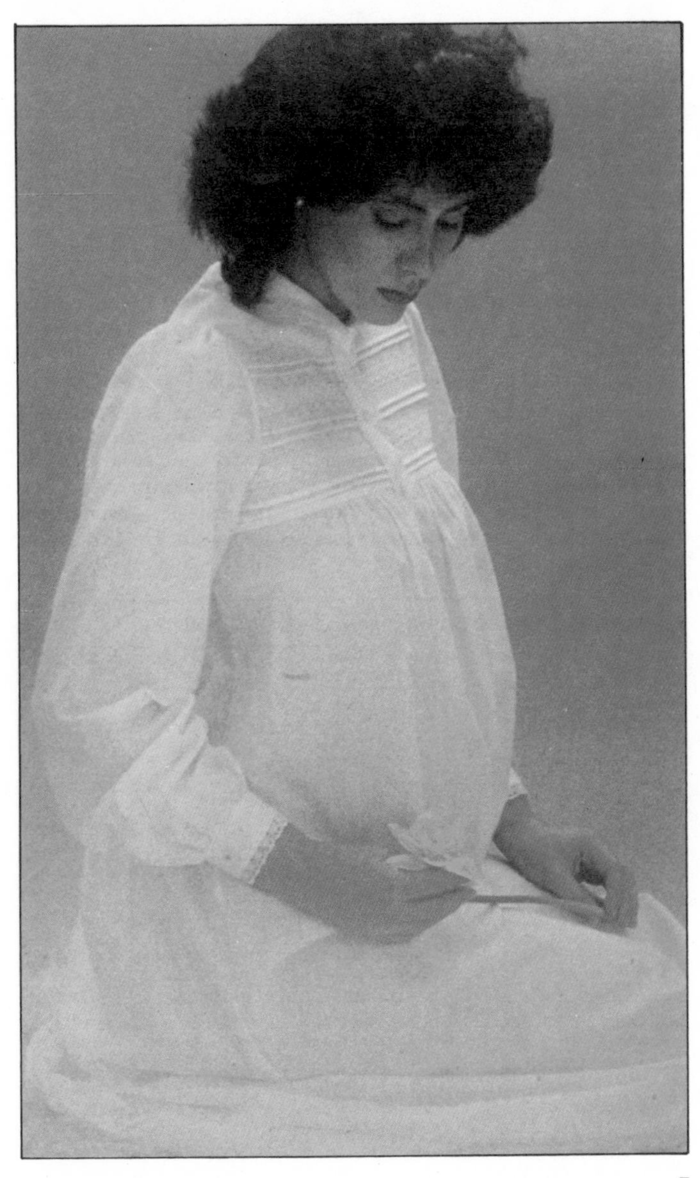

DETERMINING YOUR DUE DATE

When determining your due date, it is helpful if you have been keeping a record of the date your periods begin each month. Then, when you find you are pregnant, it will help eliminate some of the guesswork about your due date if you have this information handy on your calendar.

The average time of gestation (from conception to full term) is 266 days, although it may be as short as 240 days or as long as 300 days. Officially, that's 40 weeks, but nature rarely obeys official rules—in fact, less than five percent of all babies arrive promptly at 40 weeks.

To figure out your due date, take the first day of your last period, count back three months and add seven days. This equals nine months and seven days, or 280 days. For example, if the starting date of your last period was June 25, your due date is April 1.

If you have periods every 21 days, your baby will probably arrive a little earlier than your official due date. If your periods are on a 28-day cycle, your baby may make its appearance a little later than expected.

Determining Your Delivery Date

January	**1**	**2**	**3**	**4**	**5**	**6**	**7**	**8**	**9**	**10**	**11**	**12**	**13**	**14**	**15**	**16**	**17**	**18**	**19**	**20**	**21**	**22**	**23**	**24**	**25**	**26**	**27**	**28**	**29**	**30**	**31**
October	8	9	10	11	12	13	14	15	16	17	18	19	20	21	22	23	24	25	26	27	28	29	30	31	1	2	3	4	5	6	7
February	**1**	**2**	**3**	**4**	**5**	**6**	**7**	**8**	**9**	**10**	**11**	**12**	**13**	**14**	**15**	**16**	**17**	**18**	**19**	**20**	**21**	**22**	**23**	**24**	**25**	**26**	**27**	**28**	**29**		
November	8	9	10	11	12	13	14	15	16	17	18	19	20	21	22	23	24	25	26	27	28	29	30	1	2	3	4	5	6		
March	**1**	**2**	**3**	**4**	**5**	**6**	**7**	**8**	**9**	**10**	**11**	**12**	**13**	**14**	**15**	**16**	**17**	**18**	**19**	**20**	**21**	**22**	**23**	**24**	**25**	**26**	**27**	**28**	**29**	**30**	**31**
December	6	7	8	9	10	11	12	13	14	15	16	17	18	19	20	21	22	23	24	25	26	27	28	29	30	31	1	2	3	4	5
April	**1**	**2**	**3**	**4**	**5**	**6**	**7**	**8**	**9**	**10**	**11**	**12**	**13**	**14**	**15**	**16**	**17**	**18**	**19**	**20**	**21**	**22**	**23**	**24**	**25**	**26**	**27**	**28**	**29**	**30**	
January	6	7	8	9	10	11	12	13	14	15	16	17	18	19	20	21	22	23	24	25	26	27	28	29	30	31	1	2	3	4	
May	**1**	**2**	**3**	**4**	**5**	**6**	**7**	**8**	**9**	**10**	**11**	**12**	**13**	**14**	**15**	**16**	**17**	**18**	**19**	**20**	**21**	**22**	**23**	**24**	**25**	**26**	**27**	**28**	**29**	**30**	**31**
February	5	6	7	8	9	10	11	12	13	14	15	16	17	18	19	20	21	22	23	24	25	26	27	28	1	2	3	4	5	6	7
June	**1**	**2**	**3**	**4**	**5**	**6**	**7**	**8**	**9**	**10**	**11**	**12**	**13**	**14**	**15**	**16**	**17**	**18**	**19**	**20**	**21**	**22**	**23**	**24**	**25**	**26**	**27**	**28**	**29**	**30**	
March	8	9	10	11	12	13	14	15	16	17	18	19	20	21	22	23	24	25	26	27	28	29	30	31	1	2	3	4	5	6	
July	**1**	**2**	**3**	**4**	**5**	**6**	**7**	**8**	**9**	**10**	**11**	**12**	**13**	**14**	**15**	**16**	**17**	**18**	**19**	**20**	**21**	**22**	**23**	**24**	**25**	**26**	**27**	**28**	**29**	**30**	**31**
April	7	8	9	10	11	12	13	14	15	16	17	18	19	20	21	22	23	24	25	26	27	28	29	30	1	2	3	4	5	6	7
August	**1**	**2**	**3**	**4**	**5**	**6**	**7**	**8**	**9**	**10**	**11**	**12**	**13**	**14**	**15**	**16**	**17**	**18**	**19**	**20**	**21**	**22**	**23**	**24**	**25**	**26**	**27**	**28**	**29**	**30**	**31**
May	8	9	10	11	12	13	14	15	16	17	18	19	20	21	22	23	24	25	26	27	28	29	30	31	1	2	3	4	5	6	7
September	**1**	**2**	**3**	**4**	**5**	**6**	**7**	**8**	**9**	**10**	**11**	**12**	**13**	**14**	**15**	**16**	**17**	**18**	**19**	**20**	**21**	**22**	**23**	**24**	**25**	**26**	**27**	**28**	**29**	**30**	
June	8	9	10	11	12	13	14	15	16	17	18	19	20	21	22	23	24	25	26	27	28	29	30	1	2	3	4	5	6	7	
October	**1**	**2**	**3**	**4**	**5**	**6**	**7**	**8**	**9**	**10**	**11**	**12**	**13**	**14**	**15**	**16**	**17**	**18**	**19**	**20**	**21**	**22**	**23**	**24**	**25**	**26**	**27**	**28**	**29**	**30**	**31**
July	8	9	10	11	12	13	14	15	16	17	18	19	20	21	22	23	24	25	26	27	28	29	30	31	1	2	3	4	5	6	7
November	**1**	**2**	**3**	**4**	**5**	**6**	**7**	**8**	**9**	**10**	**11**	**12**	**13**	**14**	**15**	**16**	**17**	**18**	**19**	**20**	**21**	**22**	**23**	**24**	**25**	**26**	**27**	**28**	**29**	**30**	
August	8	9	10	11	12	13	14	15	16	17	18	19	20	21	22	23	24	25	26	27	28	29	30	31	1	2	3	4	5	6	
December	**1**	**2**	**3**	**4**	**5**	**6**	**7**	**8**	**9**	**10**	**11**	**12**	**13**	**14**	**15**	**16**	**17**	**18**	**19**	**20**	**21**	**22**	**23**	**24**	**25**	**26**	**27**	**28**	**29**	**30**	**31**
August	7	8	9	10	11	12	13	14	15	16	17	18	19	20	21	22	23	24	25	26	27	28	29	30	1	2	3	4	5	6	7

Month

Medical appointments:

Questions to ask:

Things to do this month:

Weight: Blood Pressure:

KEEPING A PREGNANCY DIARY

Pregnancy is a marvelous, unique experience. Keeping a diary during your pregnancy will help you record all the elation and joy of those nine months. A diary can serve several valuable purposes. By recording the changes in your body, your emotions, and your relationships, it will help you remember the happy times and come to terms with your moments of doubt. If you become pregnant again later, you may find it helpful to look back on the progress of the previous pregnancy. And lastly, when you look back through the pages of your diary some time in the future, you will relive the joy of that special time.

An easy way to keep a pregnancy diary is to buy a small, inexpensive, pretty notebook with at least fifty pages. Simply start each month with a new page, and then start another new page for each week of the month. Of course, you should write just as much or as little as you want—spill over onto the next page, the page after that, and even a new notebook if you like!

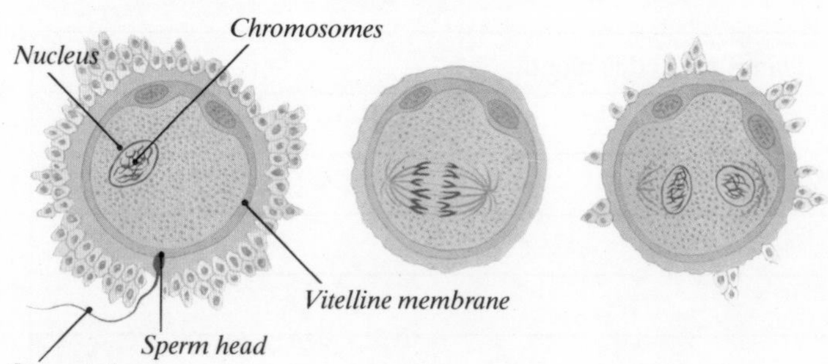

The moment of conception, *the fertilization of the female ovum by the male sperm, is the first biological event in pregnancy. A single sperm penetrates the vitelline membrane of the ovum, losing its body and tail, but keeps its head.*

The sperm nucleus, *located in the sperm head, fuses with the ovum nucleus, still high up in the fallopian tube. The chromosomes from each nucleus intermingle and pair with their opposite numbers from the other nucleus.*

The chromosomes *duplicate and separate before the first cell division of the new embryo's life. Cell division continues in the embryo as it travels down the fallopian tube towards the uterus where it implants itself about a week after fertilization, and develops into the fetus.*

Month: Week #
Monday the
Tuesday the
Wednesday the
Thursday the
Friday the
Saturday the
Sunday the

MONTH-BY-MONTH COUNTDOWN

FIRST MONTH

- It's time to start doing your homework. Buy or borrow some good, recent books on pregnancy and childbirth, and read them carefully.
- Based on your reading, your personal preferences, and your medical situation, consider the childbirth options available to you.

SECOND MONTH

- Check out your benefits. What does your company health insurance cover? Are you entitled to maternity leave, and what are the details? And what about paternity leave? What other health insurance coverage do you have, either through company or private policies or through government assistance?
- If you work, think about how and when to tell your superiors and co-workers about your pregnancy.

THIRD MONTH

- Start doing your Kegel exercises every day.
- Enroll in an exercise class designed for pregnant women.

FOURTH MONTH

- Now's the time to look into childbirth classes, even though you won't start attending until your seventh month.
- Now's also the time to start shopping for maternity clothes. You probably won't need them for another month or so, but it's easier and less fatiguing to do the shopping now.
- Keep doing your exercises!

FIFTH MONTH

- Keep doing your exercises!
- You'll start to notice real weight gain now. It's normal—so don't try to slim, but continue to eat a well-balanced diet.

SIXTH MONTH

- Keep doing your exercises!
- Keep eating! A well-balanced diet is essential for the baby's development and your own health.
- As you approach the start of the third and final trimester, try to get all major tasks—for example, painting the nursery—out of the way. If you're planning to move, do it now.

Seventh Month

- It's time to start childbirth classes.
- Keep doing your exercises and eating properly!
- Many women plan to leave their jobs during this month. If you do, make a list of all the people to notify and steps to take regarding maternity leave and so on.

Eighth Month

- Keep doing your exercises and eating properly!
- Visit the place where you will give birth, including the delivery and aftercare areas. Introduce yourself to the staff and get to know where everything is—including the pay phones and men's restrooms. When you're in labor is not the time to be exploring.
- Choose a pediatrician.
- If at all possible, arrange for help at home for the first week or so after the baby is born. A friend, relative, or professional baby nurse can really make a difference during that exhausting but important first week.
- Do you still need things for the baby or the baby's room? Get them now.
- If you plan to breast-feed, begin preparing your breasts (see "Breast-feeding").

Ninth Month

- Pack your hospital bag (see "What to Take to the Hospital").
- Pick the baby's godparents.
- Make a list of everyone you'll want to call from the hospital—and start saving change for the pay phones!
- Make a list of everyone you'll want to send a birth announcement to, and start addressing the envelopes.
- Cook and freeze some meals in advance—this can be a big help to you and your family while you're at the hospital and just after you come home.
- Relax!

MORNING SICKNESS

Morning sickness may be the first indication that you are pregnant. There are lots of jokes about it, but if you're suffering, there's nothing funny about it. Morning sickness is sudden nausea and can occur at any time of the day, although most commonly it occurs in the morning hours. Unless it becomes very severe, morning sickness has no effect on your baby.

Get plenty of fresh air in the room where you sleep and as you cook breakfast. Odors may upset your stomach. Have some dry bread or cereal by your bedside to eat before you lift your head from the pillow. Do *not* use butter or margarine (fats and greasy foods tend to upset the stomach). Get up very slowly, taking five or six minutes. Avoid sudden movements when you're feeling nauseated.

Eat several small meals a day, instead of three large ones, because you are more likely to feel nauseated when your stomach is empty. Carbonated beverages and grapefruit, orange, or grape juice may help settle your stomach. Lying down after eating may also help.

If you haven't quit smoking by now, morning sickness may be the incentive you need. Giving up cigarettes will ease your nausea —and increase the chance of having a healthy baby.

And remember, morning sickness usually passes with the end of the first trimester.

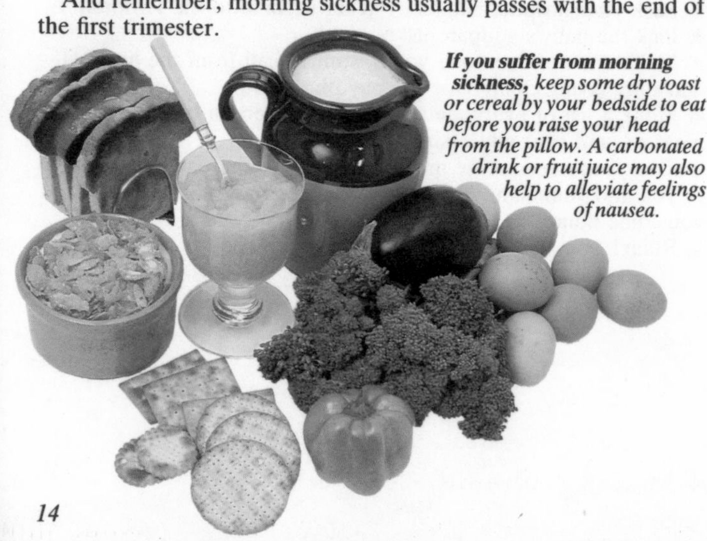

If you suffer from morning sickness, *keep some dry toast or cereal by your bedside to eat before you raise your head from the pillow. A carbonated drink or fruit juice may also help to alleviate feelings of nausea.*

ACHES AND PAINS

Pregnancy is a wonderful time, and you will experience marvelous periods of tremendous well-being. However, your body is also changing to accommodate a rapidly growing baby, and you will experience some normal aches and pains.

GROIN PAINS

A mild, achy feeling on one or both sides of your stomach is most likely due to the stretching of the ligaments around your growing uterus. As long as these pains are mild, they are nothing to worry about. They usually occur during the first three to five months of pregnancy. However, any pains that are severe in any way or feel like menstrual cramps should be reported to your doctor or midwife at once.

BRAXTON HICKS CONTRACTIONS

Toward the end of your second trimester you will probably start having occasional contractions of the uterus. These are called Braxton Hicks contractions, and they are a perfectly normal part of pregnancy—they are a sort of warm-up for the real thing, and they strengthen the uterus. Some women barely feel Braxton Hicks contractions, and others may have the cramps every ten minutes for an hour at a time. The contractions feel exactly like labor pains, but they do not get more intense, frequent, or closer together. To relieve the discomfort, try shifting your position or walking around a bit. The breathing techniques you learn in childbirth class will also help.

HEMORRHOIDS

Hemorrhoids are a common complaint of pregnancy and are the equivalent of varicose veins in your legs: they are caused by increased pressure on your veins, in this case the veins in your anus.

Constipation is the most frequent reason for the development of hemorrhoids. If you have hemorrhoids you should sit on hard, firm surfaces. Cold compresses with witch hazel may also relieve the itching and pain.

BODY TEMPERATURE

While you are pregnant your body temperature should not go too high. If you get sick and have a fever, and your temperature goes up, call the doctor or midwife immediately. He or she may prescribe acetaminophen, fluids, and bed rest.

Incidentally, this rule means staying out of hot tubs and the like.

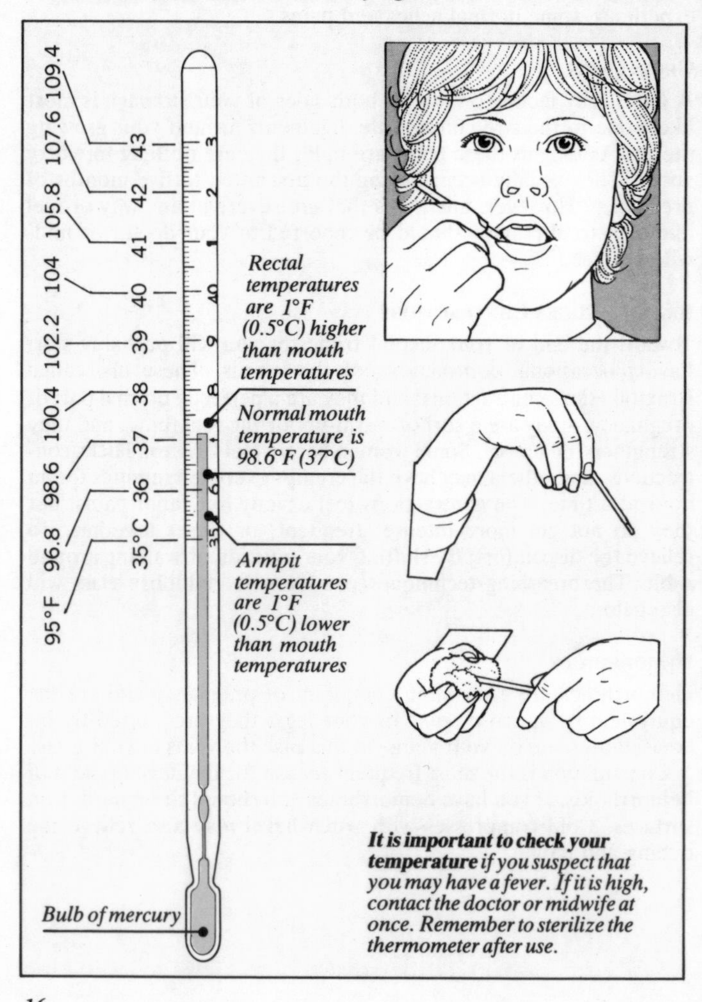

***It is important to check your temperature** if you suspect that you may have a fever. If it is high, contact the doctor or midwife at once. Remember to sterilize the thermometer after use.*

VARICOSE VEINS

The bad news is that varicose veins are ugly, bluish, worm-like veins on your legs, and are characteristic of pregnancy. The good news is that they fade after the baby is born. If your mother had them, you probably will too.

Varicose veins have two general causes (besides being hereditary): your circulation has to deal with an increased amount of fluid in your body, and your growing uterus is putting more pressure on the veins in your legs.

There are steps you can take to minimize varicose veins. Don't were "knee highs"—stockings with elastic bands along the top which stop just below your knee. In fact, don't wear any kind of stocking that cuts off circulation along any part of your leg. Support hose are expensive compared to regular pantyhose, but worth it if you tend toward varicose veins.

Elevate your legs whenever possible, and don't sit in any one position for too long. Walk and exercise as much as possible. You should also rig up a way to elevate your legs while you're sleeping, such as raising the foot of your bed slightly by placing wooden blocks underneath.

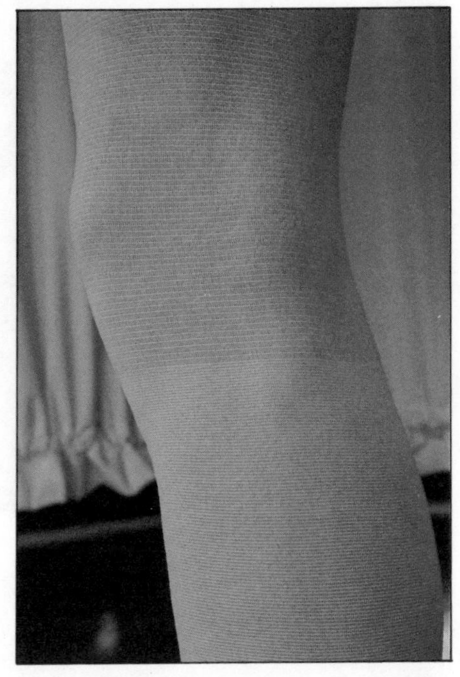

***Support stockings** may be advisable to help ease the symptoms of varicose veins — a common problem of pregnancy, but one that usually lessens after the baby is born.*

STRETCH MARKS

You may notice red, angry-looking stretch marks (striae) on various parts of your body as your skin stretches to fit your blossoming dimensions. The most common area for stretch marks is the stomach, since that is doing the most stretching as the baby grows. Your breasts, buttocks, and thighs may also get stretch marks.

The good news is that stretch marks will eventually fade to become white, silvery lines. When tanned they will not be as noticeable. The bad news is that the jury is still out regarding the prevention of stretch marks.

There are various theories and remedies for the "cure" of stretch marks. The most common is that rubbing cream, particularly coconut-oil–based concoctions, into the skin will help it become more elastic and thus resistant to marks. Some medical opinion scoffs at this remedy, however, arguing that there's nothing you can put on the surface of the skin to lessen a function that is going on below the top layer.

In any case, applying cream to the area will help ease the itching caused by your stretching skin. Your partner, who may quite often feel helpless in the face of your discomfort, can also assist by applying the cream for you.

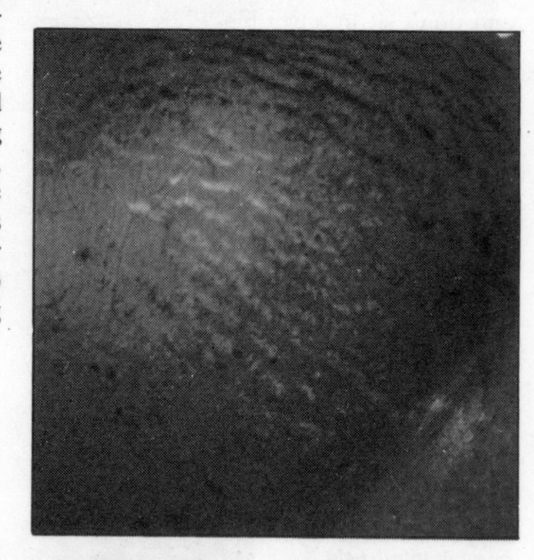

About one third of pregnant women develop stretch marks *as their body expands with the growing fetus. Apart from the lower stomach, stretch marks may also appear on the breasts, buttocks and thighs.*

CONSTIPATION

Constipation is a very common complaint of pregnant women. It's not very funny and it's not very pleasant. During pregnancy bowels are more sluggish, and less efficient. The iron supplement your doctor may prescribe as part of your prenatal vitamin intake might also cause constipation.

Being "regular" doesn't necessarily mean a bowel movement every day. And don't strain—you'll only end up with hemorrhoids, which aren't very pleasant either. The definition of constipation is the passing of a hard stool—and if you do this all day long, you're still technically constipated.

There are remedies however: eat fresh fruit and green vegetables, and drink lots of fluids. Some people swear by hot lemon water three times a day, others say a little licorice candy can help. Exercise, even if it's just walking, will also help stimulate the bowel. All of the above (with the exception of the licorice candy) are also good for you, pregnant or not.

Metamucil is a natural bulk laxative with no chemical additives. You can use it as often as you need to. Establishing a regular time for moving your bowels, and elevating your feet on a footstool while sitting on the toilet, may also help.

Fresh fruit and vegetables, *which are high in fiber, are a natural remedy for constipation.*

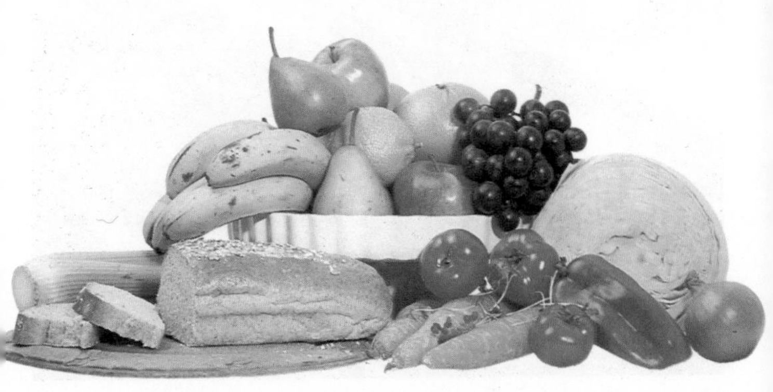

INDIGESTION AND GAS

Indigestion, which most often manifests itself as heartburn, in pregnant women is caused by food remaining longer than usual in the stomach. The good thing about this is that the nutrients in the food are absorbed better. But the bad thing is that you may feel awfully uncomfortable, especially toward the end of your pregnancy.

Most pregnant women get heartburn at some time or other, usually in the final trimester. Don't eat spicy or greasy foods, the

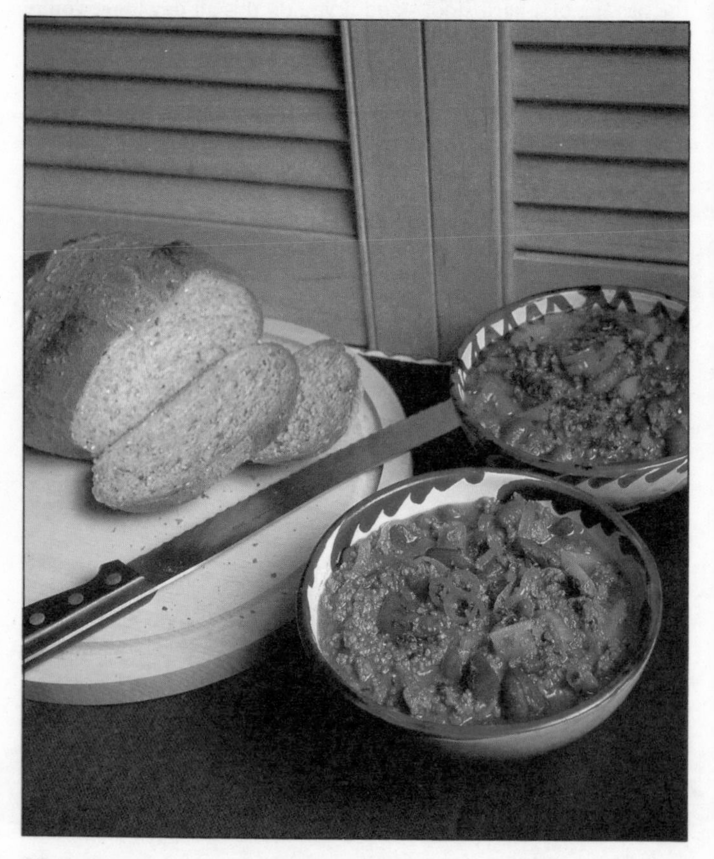

most common cause of heartburn. Toward the end of their pregnancy many women find themselves eating nothing but plain rice and flavored gelatine. If the problem gets really uncomfortable, talk to your doctor or midwife about it.

Try drinking milk with your meal, since it coats your stomach.

You could also try eating several small meals a day. Large meals will make you feel bloated and aggravate your indigestion.

Gas

Gas (flatulence) is another embarrassing problem of pregnancy. You'll notice you feel like an urpy, burpy, gassy lady almost as soon as you get pregnant.

There is a very real reason for gas in pregnant women: your stomach and intestines are distended, so that bloated feeling is very real.

There is unfortunately no cure for gas. Try to have a sense of humor about it. There are, however, several things you can do to try to lessen gas: have regular bowel movements, eat puréed vegetables to increase intestinal activity, and avoid foods that produce gas like beans, cabbage, fried foods, and so on.

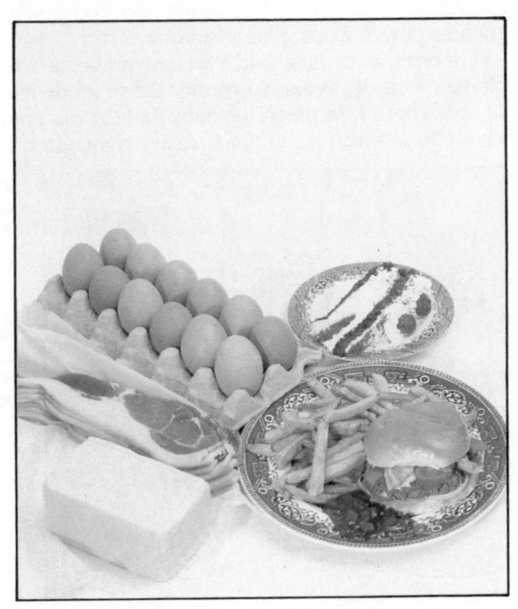

***Pulses** (left) may aggravate a tendency toward flatulence and should be avoided if gas is a problem.*

***Greasy foods,** such as hamburger and french fries (right) or fried eggs and bacon, are a common cause of heartburn.*

WEIGHT GAIN

Being thin is a national fixation. Consequently, one of the most difficult adjustments for many pregnant women is that they are going to gain weight and that this weight gain (within reason) is a good thing.

You know, on an intellectual level, that you are growing a baby inside of you and that is why you are gaining weight. But many women feel devastated with every additional pound, so conditioned are they by what "fashion" dictates. You may feel ugly, unfeminine, and unloved. The result is that you'll feel guilty, resentful, and constantly worried. This is hard on you, hard on your baby, and hard on your partner, who must listen to your unending complaints and constantly try to reassure you.

The weight you gain is good. It provides protection and nurturance for your baby. This doesn't mean you can comfort yourself every day with a huge ice cream sundae: you're eating for two in terms of nutrition, not quantity. You have to consume more calories to feed the developing fetus, but this doesn't entitle you to munch away happily on anything and everything—empty calories such as potato chips benefit no one.

Theories as to how much weight pregnant women should gain change with the years. Currently, 25 to 35 pounds is the accepted figure. That's how much the baby and the placenta weigh, so that's about how much you'll lose easily right after the baby is born

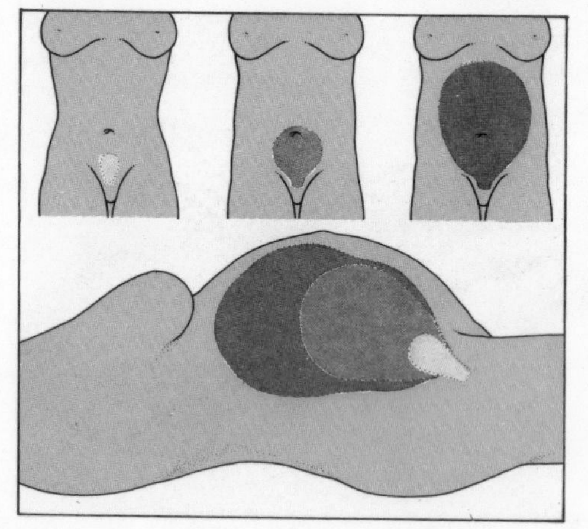

***The growth of the uterus** at 12, 25 and 36 weeks of pregnancy (left). Weight gain is most marked during the fifth and sixth month, and by the end of the third trimester the baby and placenta weigh, on average, 25 to 35 pounds. Following a well-balanced diet (right) will ensure that surplus weight gain is kept to a minimum.*

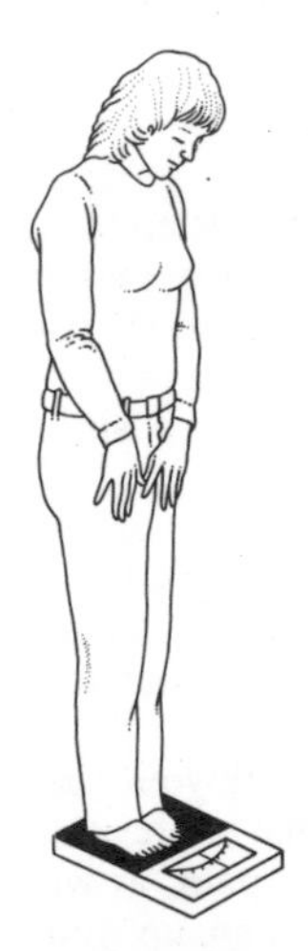

***Keep a weekly record of your weight gain** and report any change in the pattern to your doctor.*

(you'll lose approximately 12 pounds as an immediate result of the delivery). Anything more than that, says the conventional wisdom, and you'll have to work hard to get it off. And dieting is never, ever, anything more than a bore.

However, don't be dominated or bullied about your weight. Certainly gross obesity or scrawny thinness is not good for you or for your baby, but if you gain more than 25 pounds, don't feel guilty. Everybody is different; every pregnancy is different. The important thing is the rate at which you gain weight: it should be steady and consistent, with the most gain taking place in the fifth and sixth month. You should keep a weekly weigh-in record, and report any weight loss or change in the pattern of weight gain to your doctor.

And don't starve yourself on the day before your regular visit to the doctor. This may make your chart look good, but you are depriving your baby of food, and that is not a very good idea.

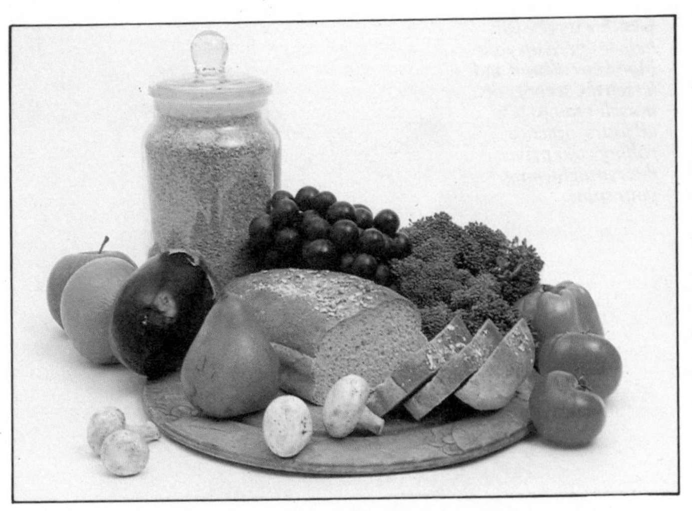

MUSCLE CRAMPS

Muscle cramps in your legs and feet are an unpleasant side effect of pregnancy. Many sleepless nights are the result of a nasty muscle cramp. Cramps are the result of slower blood circulation. (If you experience shooting pains in your legs, it could be due to a pinched nerve thanks to the pressure of the baby's head. Shift your position to relieve it.)

There are several counter-measures you can employ to ensure you don't get muscle cramps (or to lessen their frequency). Don't point your toes while exercising. Take an increased level of calcium and potassium, with your doctor's permission. Elevate your legs while sleeping.

Once you get a cramp, straighten your leg by forcing your toes up toward your chin and pushing your knee down flat. A heating pad or hot-water bottle will help relieve the residual pain, as will massage. Since your agony will probably have woken up your partner, perhaps he can do these things for you.

Menstrual-like cramps in your abdomen should be reported to your doctor *immediately*. They can be a serious sign of possible miscarriage. You should not experience menstrual cramps in your abdomen at any time during your pregnancy.

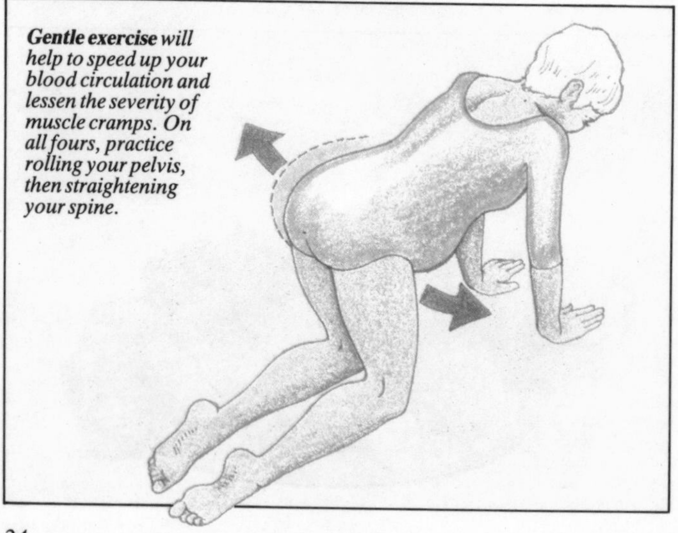

***Gentle exercise** will help to speed up your blood circulation and lessen the severity of muscle cramps. On all fours, practice rolling your pelvis, then straightening your spine.*

SWELLING

Swelling, also known as edema, is a normal part of pregnancy. It is caused by water retention due to an increase in the female hormones necessary to build the placenta.

Swollen ankles are usually the first sign that you have edema. Swollen hands and fingers are another sign. Your breasts may also throb as they swell with the increase in milk gland activity. The net result is that you may feel terribly bloated and you may fear a heart attack is imminent, but neither is actually the case.

It doesn't help to know that edema is typical of pregnancy—the swelling only serves to make you feel even fatter. However, excessive swelling is not normal and should be reported to your doctor—it could be a sign of pre-eclampsia or eclampsia (toxemia of pregnancy).

Women who are pregnant during the hot summer months will experience more swelling of ankles and hands. Wear loose-fitting clothes and remove your rings if your hands swell.

Don't stand for long periods — elevate your feet above your hips as often as possible. Exercise such as walking helps, and so does cutting out salty foods (you need some salt, though). If you eat more protein, it will help absorb the water in your body.

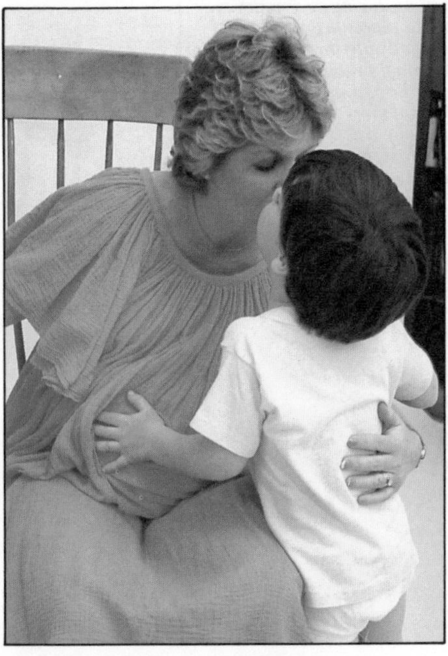

***Water retention** in pregnancy results in swelling — most commonly of the ankles, hands and fingers. To alleviate symptoms, take the weight off your feet by frequently sitting down.*

BLEEDING

You should never bleed from your vagina while you are pregnant. If you do start to bleed, even a small amount, *notify your doctor or midwife at once.*

Apart from the "bloody show" (discussed elsewhere) that signals the onset of labor, bleeding in the final three months of your pregnancy is especially serious and may mean a possibly life-threatening situation for you and the baby, such as placenta previa. This is a condition where the placenta is covering the cervix, which is the baby's exit. If you know from an earlier ultrasound test that your placenta is in the wrong place, go immediately to the hospital if you start bleeding. Tell the attending doctor of your probable condition. Don't let anyone outside of the hospital (such as a doctor or paramedic in an ambulance) do any kind of internal exam on you, as this can worsen the possible hemorrhage.

***Bleeding during pregnancy** may indicate placenta previa, a potentially life-threatening situation for mother and baby in which the placenta covers the mouth of the womb. Because swift diagnosis is essential, any blood loss, however small, must be reported at once.*

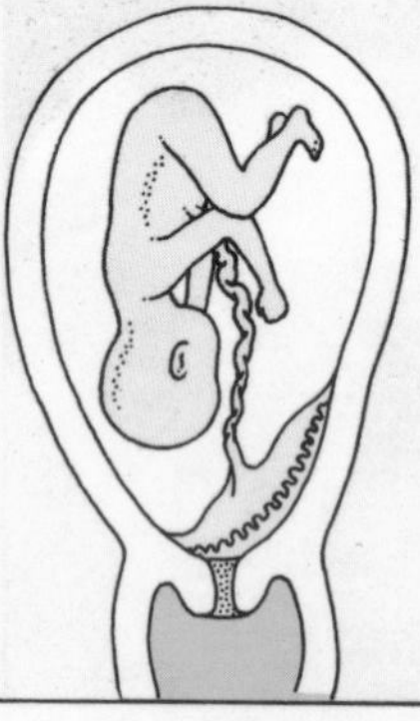

BACKACHE

Backache is almost a certainty with pregnancy. And it's caused by a very simple thing: you are carrying a heavier weight. But you don't have to suffer in silence—there are several remedies to help relieve backache.

Good posture is especially important: sit up straight with good lower back support, and stand up straight with your bottom and your hips tucked under and your stomach tipped in as far as possible. Arching your back when you stand or walk will only aggravate the ache of your lower back region.

Change your position frequently. If your work is primarily sitting at a desk, get up and move around as often as possible. Use a footstool and alternate shifting your weight from one leg to another (your knees should be just slightly higher than your hips).

If your job involves long periods of standing, lean forward or bend your knees slightly sometimes. Or lean on a table top or similar surface and place your weight on your hands or elbows. This takes your weight off your back.

Exercise also helps backache. Talk to your doctor about suitable exercises. One frequently used movement is called the pelvic rock: kneel on your hands and knees, elbows and back straight, knees slightly apart. Arch your back up like a hissing cat while you inhale and tuck your chin down on your chest. Slowly exhale and relax. Use your lower stomach muscles to arch your back up.

Another helpful exercise is to get on your hands and knees and pull one knee into your chest while tucking your chin down, so the knee touches (or nearly touches) your chin. Straighten out your neck and extend your leg straight out behind you at the same time.

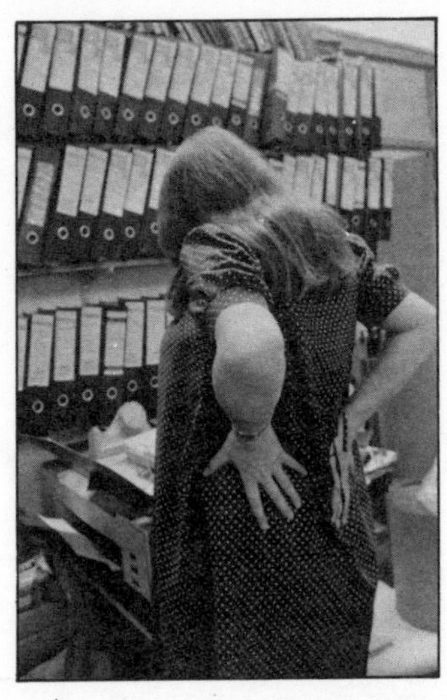

***Backache can rarely be avoided during pregnancy**. If your job involves sitting at a desk, get up periodically to stretch your legs.*

Correct lifting and carrying while you are pregnant are also important. (See other sections of this book for more information.)
Massage or a heating pad can help relieve backache, and both are something your partner can help you with.

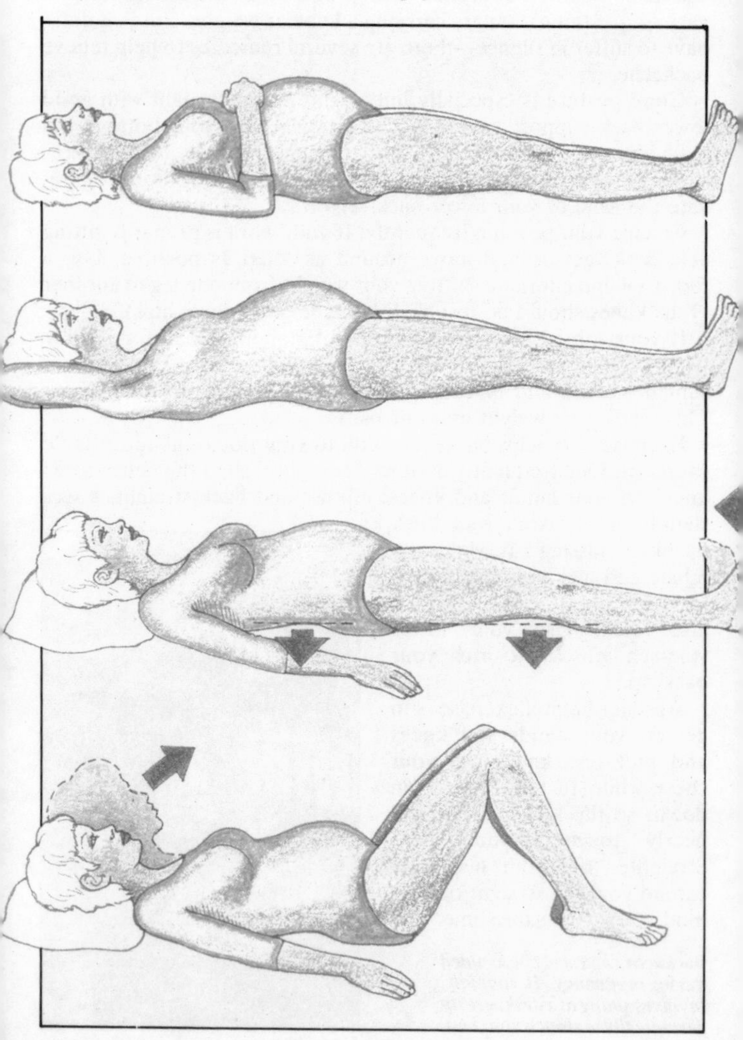

POSTURE

In order to maintain balance and decrease fatigue and backache, you should learn to adapt your posture and body movement to the changes in weight and increased pressures that pregnancy causes.

Here are some rules to live by:

- Avoid bending from the waist; always bend your hips and knees at the same time.
- Avoid lifting heavy objects higher than your waist.
- Always turn and face the object you wish to lift.
- Avoid carrying unbalanced loads.
- Never carry or move anything you cannot handle easily.
- Avoid sudden movements. Learn to move slowly.
- Change positions frequently. Balance periods of activity with rest.
- Avoid exercises that arch or strain the lower back (touching toes, bending backward).
- When mopping, vacuuming, raking, hoeing, etc., always work with the tool close to your body. Keep your knees bent and back straight. Avoid "giant steps."
- Wear low heels.
- Never point your toes while stretching or exercising.
- Do not lean over the sink when washing, brushing your teeth, or doing the dishes. Lower your body by bending your knees and hips while keeping your back straight.

***Exercises that gently tone the muscles of the back** without running the risk of straining them may help to alleviate backache: lying flat on the floor (opposite, top), squeeze your buttock muscles together and tighten your stomach muscles; then try to press your back and waist "into" the floor. Hold for four seconds and relax. Still on your back (opposite, bottom), first bend and stretch your ankles, and follow by bending and straightening your knees. Finally, lift your head. Hold each movement for 10 seconds and relax.*

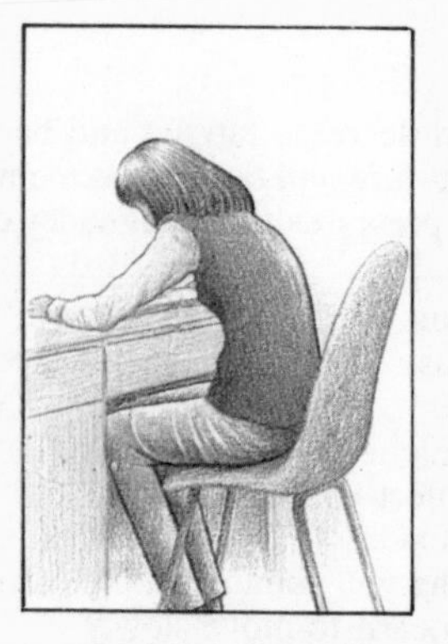

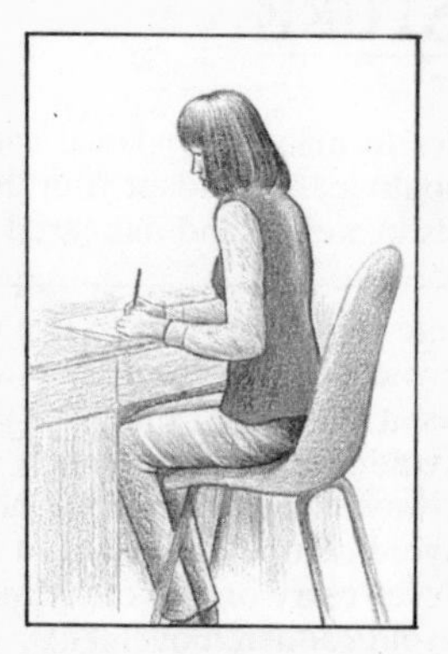

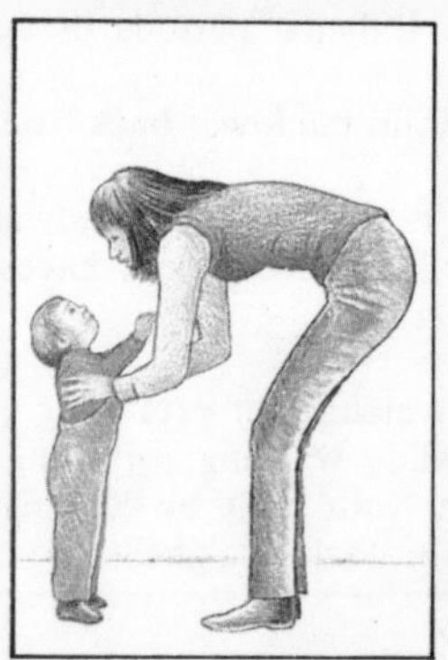

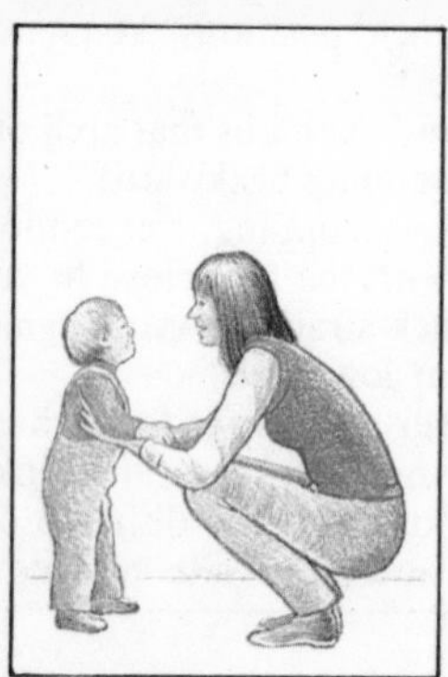

***A good posture is always important,** especially when you are pregnant. In particular take great care of your back when sitting or lifting. When sitting at a table or slaving over the sink, try not to slouch (top left), but keep your back as straight as you can (top right). Lifting incorrectly (bottom left) is a primary cause of back problems such as a slipped disk. Use your strong leg muscles to take the strain (bottom right) and keep your back as straight as possible.*

EXERCISE

Exercise is always a good idea, especially so while you are pregnant. If you maintain some sort of exercise program while you are expecting, you will reap the rewards in many ways. Physically, you will feel healthier, and will be better equipped to deal with the stress of labor and delivery (which is, after all, a major physical activity in your life). Exercise also helps the blood circulation in your body and increases the oxygen content of your blood, all of which is good news for you and for your developing baby.

Psychologically, you will also feel better for exercise. Not only will you feel less clumsy, there is also a certain innate satisfaction in feeling you are exercising well and maintaining fitness.

And, if you exercise while you are pregnant you will find the effort to return to your pre-pregnant shape less grueling after delivery. It will also help you maintain a proper weight gain during pregnancy.

There are, however, important rules to remember when exercising. Now more than ever you should definitely follow the rule of checking with your doctor before starting any exercise program. Some forms of exercise, such as aerobics or running, may be forbidden to some pregnant women for various reasons.

Whatever form of exercise you choose, it should be slow, rhythmic and non-stressful. You should never, ever, exercise to the point of physical exhaustion. Walking and swimming are particularly good exercises: walking at a brisk pace a mile or more every day can really help.

Jogging is not an especially good exercise while you are pregnant, because it strains your growing breasts and your back. You

Strenuous running *is not an ideal form of exercise when you are pregnant.*

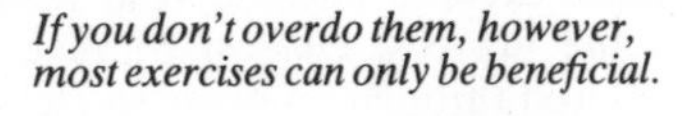

If you don't overdo them, however, most exercises can only be beneficial.

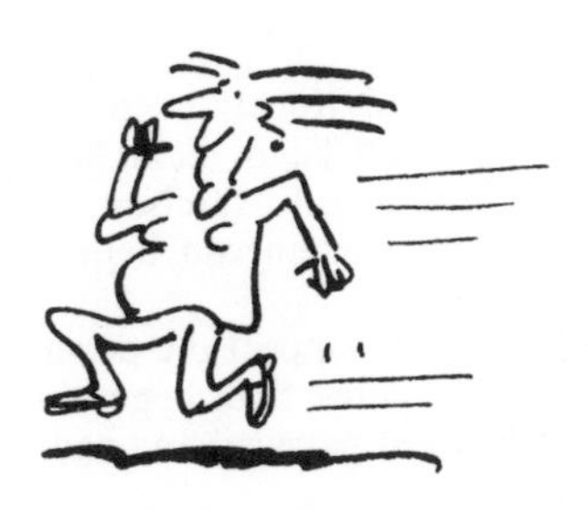

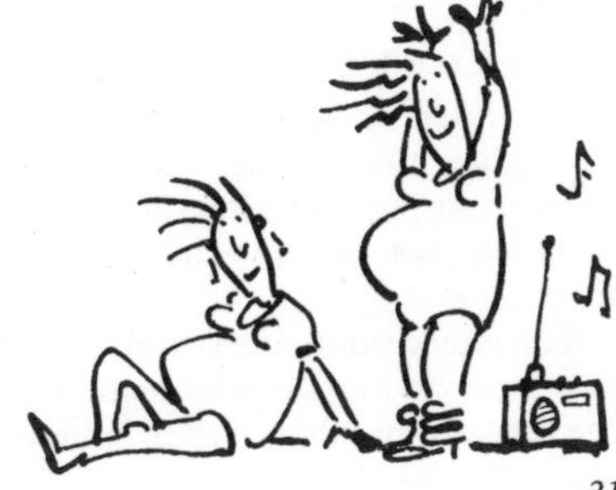

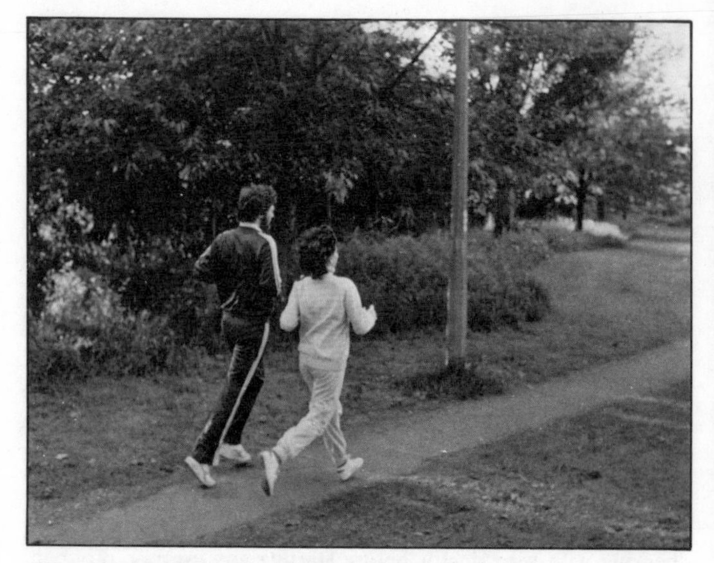

If you enjoy jogging, *it will probably do you no harm if you continue doing it carefully, so long as you don't feel uncomfortable. In particular, be careful not to strain your growing breasts and your back.*

can also cheerfully strike off sit-ups from your list. Because your uterus is expanding, the muscles on either side of your abdomen are designed to part. Doing sit-ups may cause these muscles to widen even more, making it more difficult to get back a flat tummy after you deliver.

The hospital where you plan to deliver will probably have prenatal exercise classes. Your local YMCA/YWCA may also offer some low-cost classes. More costly classes may or may not be offered through an exercise club or health spa.

Kegel Exercises

Pelvic floor or Kegel (named for Dr. Arnold Kegel) exercises strengthen the muscles of the pelvic area and keep them firm before, during and after pregnancy. In fact, Kegel exercises are definitely not just for pregnant women—all women can benefit from them.

The pelvic floor consists of muscle layers that support the pelvic organs, including the womb and bladder. The pelvic floor begins in the area around the urethral sphincter (the front passage) and ends at the rectal sphincter (the back passage). During pregnancy, this is an area that comes under a great deal of stress as the uterus grows, putting additional weight and pressure on it. The stress can cause hemorrhoids, incontinence and other problems during pregnancy; if the pelvic floor is too weak, problems such as a prolapsed uterus can develop later.

Kegel exercises help prevent those problems by strengthening the muscles. You'll also be able to relax the pelvic floor, which will be a big help during delivery.

Here's how to do Kegel exercises:

- Tighten the muscles of the front sphincter, as if you were urinating and stopping the flow. Hold them tight for a few seconds and then release.
- Tighten the vaginal muscles, hold tight for a few seconds, and then release.
- Repeat with the muscles of the back passage.
- Repeat for all three areas two or three times; repeat the entire sequence ten times a day.

At first you may have difficulty distinguishing the different sets of muscles, but you will quickly learn which is which. Kegel exercises are easy to do anywhere, any time—while stopped at a red light or watching TV, for example. Another good place to practice them is in bed with your partner—he can tell you how well you're doing.

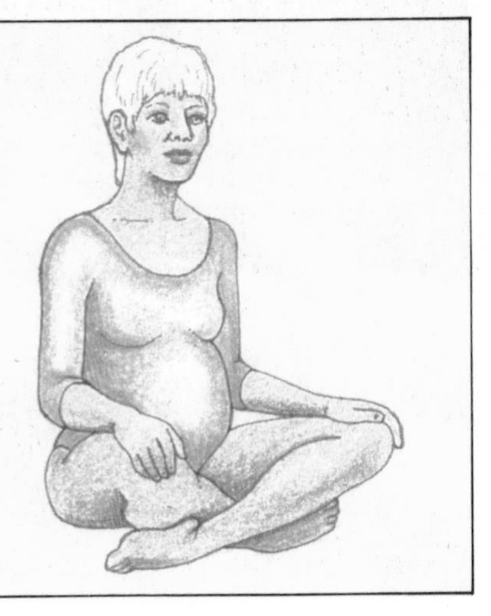

Kegel exercises can be done almost anywhere, *although you may find them most effective if you do them when sitting comfortably upright, with your legs crossed in front of you.*

FAINTING

Fainting or dizziness is not uncommon in pregnancy. Usually it is caused by blood pooling in your legs or by a drop in your blood pressure. Both are usually due to your growing uterus pressing on major blood vessels. Report any fainting or dizzy spells to your doctor.

To minimize the dizziness, move slowly and carefully. If you're an active, energetic type always hopping up and down, stop it and slow down. Change your position gradually. In particular, get up off the floor or out of a lying-down position very slowly. Faintness is often caused by standing up too quickly. So bring yourself to a sitting position, rest for a few seconds, then stand up completely.

If you find you suffer from dizziness or even fainting, *try to sit or even lie down rather than standing upright when you don't have to be moving about. This helps prevent blood pooling in your legs, which can harm the blood vessels there, and is also likely to reduce the risk of fainting, which can easily occur during pregnancy if the growing uterus presses on one of the body's major blood vessels. When you want to take exercise, try walking in the countryside or in parks where you can also rest and relax in the fresh air when you feel the need.*

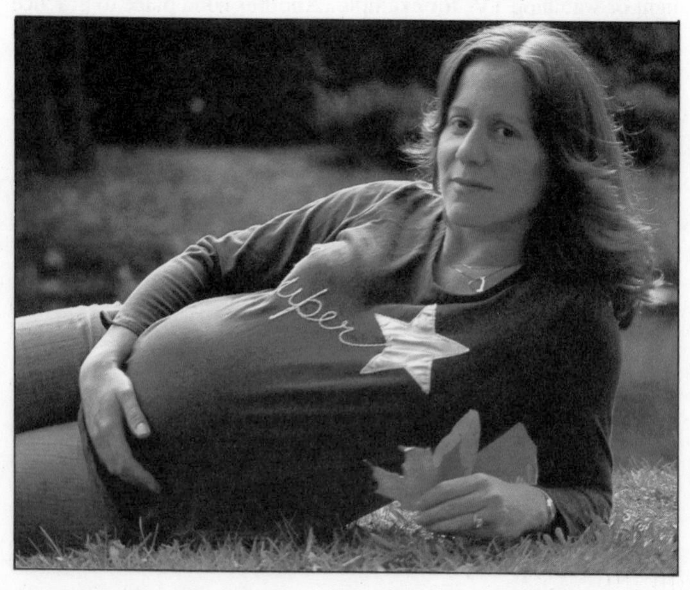

SHORTNESS OF BREATH

One of the minor discomforts (although not so minor for some!) of pregnancy is the feeling that you can't get enough air, or shortness of breath. This feeling, which can be accompanied by dizziness and faintness, is not just because you're gaining weight: there are three very good reasons for it.

Because the baby depends on your breathing for its oxygen (which it gets, as you do, through the bloodstream), you breathe deeper while you are pregnant. This isn't something you have to practice or be conscious of; you just naturally breathe deeper to accommodate the increased need for oxygen. You are literally breathing for two!

Secondly, like people who live at high altitudes, your ribcage expands. This increase in size is permanent and will not diminish even after you've lost the maternity weight gain. In fact, you may need a larger bra size even after the delivery, not because of an increase in breast size but because of your new, more robust, rib-cage. But even though you are taking in more air at a time, your lung capacity does not increase.

Finally, as your uterus grows it pushes up against the ribcage, giving you a feeling that your breathing room is crowded or tightened.

The final three months of your pregnancy are the most uncomfortable, and you will notice shortness of breath the most during this period. Try to relax and keep in mind that it is a temporary discomfort. Some women become very conscious of the need to breathe, and this ironically makes it harder to breathe. To rid yourself of the feeling that you can't breathe, or can't get enough air, walk around or change your position. Forget about your breathing —you're not going to stop breathing just because you don't concentrate on it. Another method to try is to take several deep breaths at a time (stop if you make yourself dizzy).

BREASTS AND NIPPLES

Your breasts will swell during the very earliest days of your pregnancy. This is caused by the development of the milk glands as the breasts prepare to feed the baby. If you have always been small-breasted and unhappy about that state of affairs, this may be one aspect of your blossoming figure you can rejoice over.

Unfortunately, your breasts may also feel uncomfortable, as during your periods, and tingle, hurt, or even throb. Generally, such sensitivity will lessen during the course of your pregnancy.

You may also notice a certain lumpiness. Continue to do your monthly breast-lump checks. Any lumps that are hard or dimple the skin should be reported to your doctor immediately. A technique called diaphanography, which will not harm the fetus, can be used to detect breast cancer.

Wear a support bra at all times during your pregnancy. If you have particularly large breasts it may be advisable to wear a support bra even in bed at night. Contrary to popular folklore, it isn't breast-feeding that causes droopy breasts, it's the weight gained during the very earliest months of pregnancy—wearing an adequate support bra will help prevent loss of breast tone.

Because of increased blood supply to the breasts, your veins may become more noticeable (you may also notice this on your abdomen).

The area around your nipples, called the areola, also increases in size as it darkens in color. This darker pigment will probably not disappear after the baby arrives.

You may notice a sticky, yellowish, or watery discharge from the nipples after a few months of pregnancy. This is called colostrum. It is perfectly normal and nothing to be alarmed about. In fact, if you are going to breast-feed, it will be the baby's first meal, before your real milk comes in. The color of the colostrum may change to whitish and look more like milk as you get closer to the delivery date.

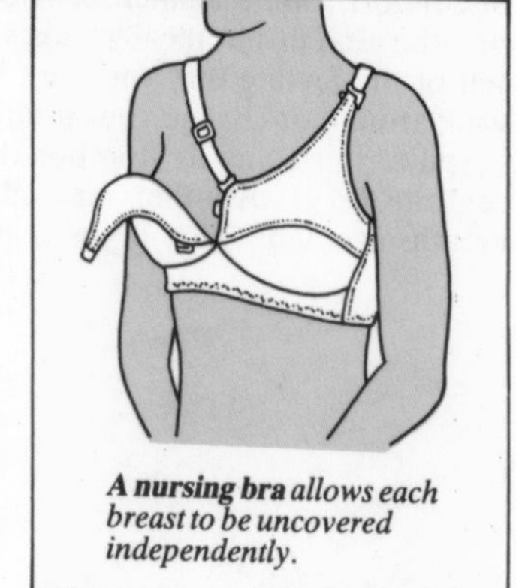

***A nursing bra** allows each breast to be uncovered independently.*

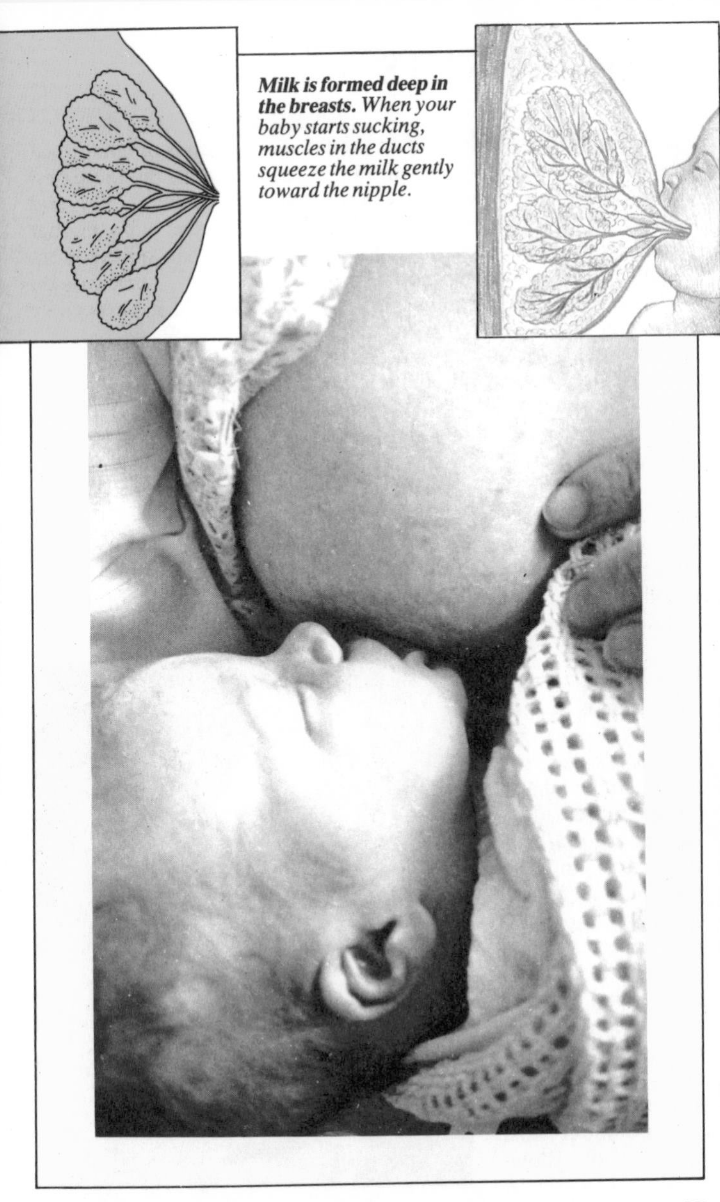

Milk is formed deep in the breasts. *When your baby starts sucking, muscles in the ducts squeeze the milk gently toward the nipple.*

HAIR AND NAILS

Many hairdressers claim they can tell that a woman is pregnant just by her hair. For nearly half of all pregnant women, the increased hormonal activity of pregnancy makes the hair thicker, shinier, and healthier. Although nobody can promise that you'll be in that happy group, you should take good care of your hair during pregnancy. In the two to six months following delivery, most women will lose some of their hair. This is unavoidable, so it's especially important to take care of your hair now.

The sudden changes in your body's hormones can cause changes in your hair. You may find the texture of your hair changing slightly —but not as drastically as it may change after you give birth. It is more likely that you'll suddenly find your hair much oilier or drier than usual.

DRY HAIR

If your hair is dry, brittle, and is developing split ends, try getting a good haircut, one that doesn't need to be blow-dried or set. Get regular trims. Use a mild shampoo every second or third day, and follow it with a good conditioner.

OILY HAIR

Your hair is getting oily if you find that it lacks body and needs to be shampooed more often. Again, a good haircut that is simple to care for is suggested. Shampoo more often with a mild shampoo. In general, you won't need a conditioner. However, if the ends of your hair are dry or split, use a conditioner just on the ends. Blow-

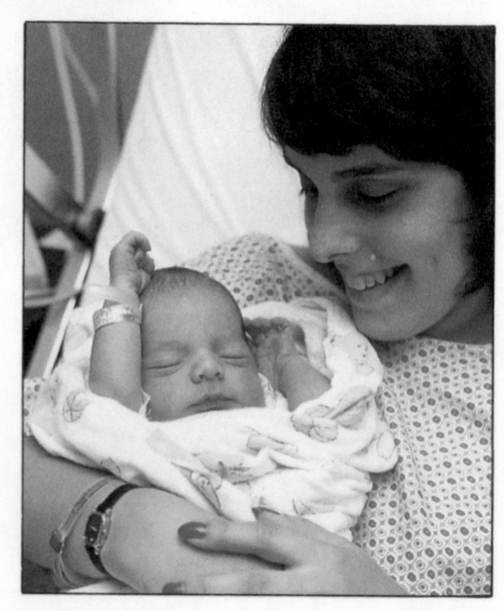

dryers and electric curlers will be fine. And remember that stress can make oily hair worse. Relax!

Hairstyles for Pregnant Women

A flattering hairstyle will help you look and feel your best while you are pregnant. Since many women become fuller in the face from weight gain, you may want to avoid pulling your hair straight back, since this makes a full face look rounder. Also avoid very long or very short styles, and avoid bangs. Perhaps the best look is a soft, simple, medium-length style with some fullness to it—cool, easy to take care of, and flattering.

Think carefully before you make a drastic change in your hairstyle. Your body is going through so many other changes that a big change in your appearance might be too much for both you and your partner.

Hair Treatments

Pregnant women should avoid hair dyes. Recent tests have demonstrated that such dyes can be carcinogenic and can enter your bloodstream—and therefore the baby's bloodstream as well.

Most women should also avoid permanents while they are pregnant. Experience has shown that for some strange reason, most hair permanents do not "take" when applied to the head of a pregnant woman. This can cause a certain amount of consternation if you've just handed over a lot of money for your usual permanent. If you can't stand straight hair while you're pregnant, cut it.

Nails

With all the calcium you're consuming (and you should be getting quite a lot to help your baby's bones build), your nails will probably take on a new, healthy beauty. Even if you've always been plagued by split or thin nails, you will probably notice that your nails are strong and healthy.

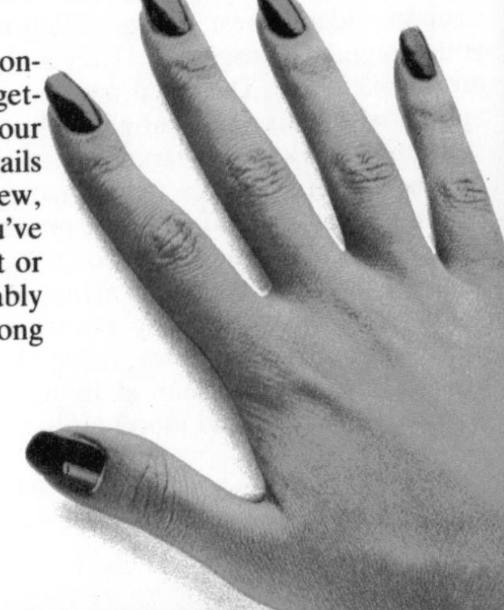

***Take special care of your nails** when you are pregnant. The changes in your body can also affect them.*

SKIN

Your skin will change during pregnancy. As with your hair, you may notice that it becomes drier or more oily. If it becomes more oily, wash with an astringent and try to avoid oil-based make-up as much as possible. If it becomes drier, lather on creams and lotions at every opportunity.

CHLOASMA

Mask of pregnancy (chloasma) is a common sign of pregnancy. It is characterized by brown spots that may appear on the face, neck, and stomach. Sometimes the spots are so extensive that a woman can appear to have a raccoon-like "mask" on her face. Chloasma appears more frequently in brunettes and black women, but any woman can have it. The spots usually appear during the second or third months, and usually fade away in about a month after delivery. Sunshine can bring on chloasma or make it worse, so avoid sunlight or wear a good sunblock.

Some black women develop areas of unpigmented skin on the face, neck and upper back. These will usually go away after delivery.

SPIDER VEINS

Two-thirds of all pregnant women will develop broken blood vessels that look like little red spiders—spider angiomas or spider nevae. These may appear on your nose or cheeks, or sometimes on your shoulders, chest, or back. You may develop more spiders as your pregnancy progresses. They are particularly noticeable if you are fair-skinned. The good news is that spider veins usually disappear within six weeks of giving birth.

Stretch marks and darkening of your nipples are two other common characteristics of pregnancy (these are discussed elsewhere in this book). If you were prone to getting pimples before or during your menstrual cycle, you will probably get them now, since some of the same hormonal action is occurring in your body.

On the good side, many women experience a "rosy glow" to their skin during pregnancy, much like your early teen years when your skin may have been at its best. Whatever the cause, be it hormonal or increased blood pressure, enjoy the radiance.

***Many women** develop a wonderfully radiant skin during pregnancy.*

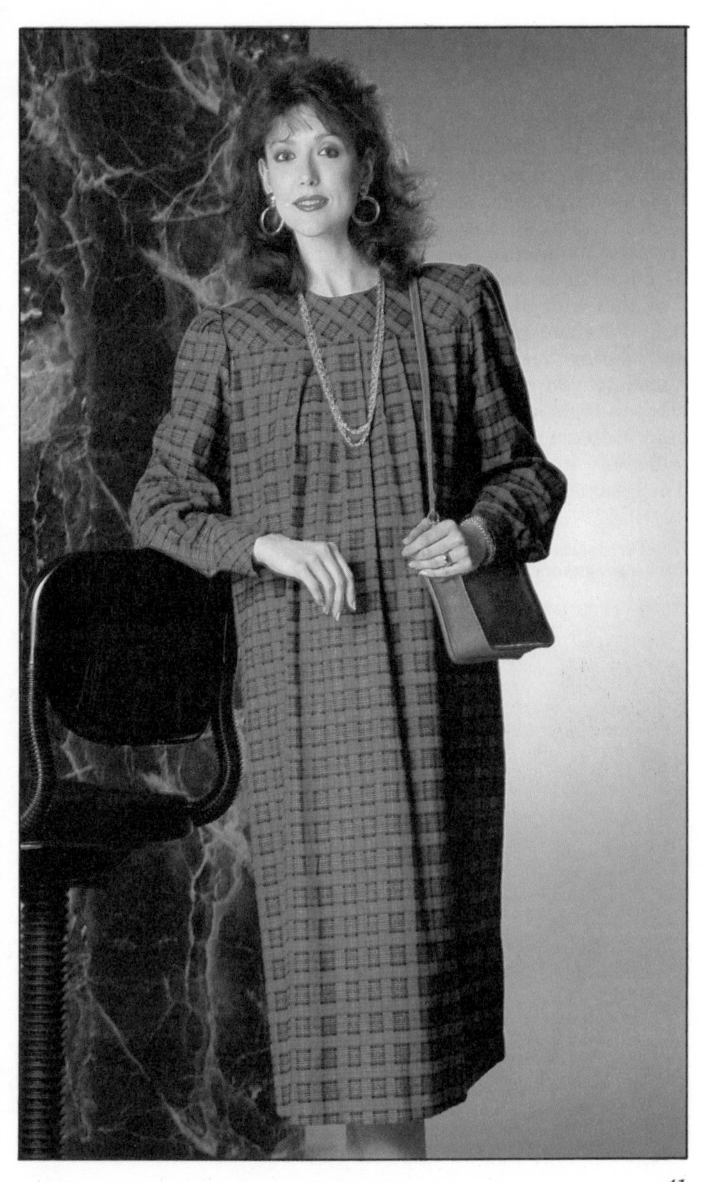

TEETH AND GUMS

There is an old wives' tale that a mother loses a tooth for every child she gives birth to. While pregnancy may affect your teeth and gums, with proper dental care you will not lose any teeth and the health of your gums should not worsen.

But because of hormonal activity your gums may be more susceptible to disease, especially your upper jaw. You may have bleeding gums, too.

A diet with the proper amounts of protein and calcium should help eliminate any problems, as will a good program of brushing and flossing. See your dentist regularly and discuss any problems or questions you have with him or her. You should have your teeth cleaned regularly by a dental hygienist, especially if you suspect a gum problem.

Be sure to tell your dentist and the staff that you are pregnant. They should not X-ray your mouth.

Good dental care is very important during pregnancy. *Hormonal changes can affect your teeth and gums, so visit your dentist regularly.*

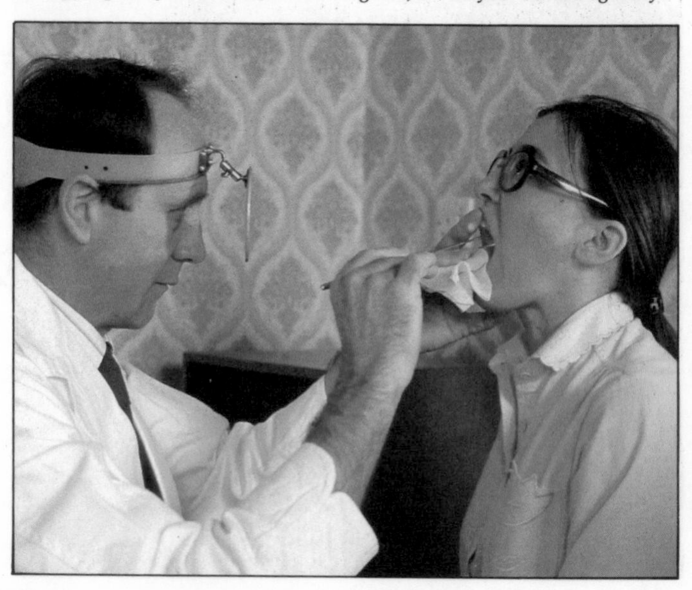

NUTRITION

Good nutrition is the single most important thing necessary for the health of you and your baby. Your doctor or midwife should provide you with a detailed diet to follow which includes all the essential vitamins and minerals you need while you are pregnant.

The amounts you are expected to eat can be daunting, especially if you're accustomed to having to fight the bulge in your life prior to pregnancy. There's no way, you think, you can eat all that and gain only 25 to 35 pounds. If that is really the case, try Weight Watchers. This organization has an excellent diet for pregnant women that allows all the right nutrients and none of the wrong empty calories. It has a good menu variety to keep you from getting bored and cheating.

Even if you're not accustomed to having to fight the bulge, you're probably far too busy to sit around writing out complex menus for yourself. Suffice it to say, the important thing is to eat regular, sensible meals.

The basic rules are that you eat the following every day: one Vitamin C food (fruit or vegetable), four servings of protein, four servings of milk (or milk products such as cheese), three servings of grain (typically bread), two leafy green vegetables and one other fruit or vegetable. Your daily intake should average about 500 calories over your pre-pregnant intake (which should have been, when not dieting, about 2,000 calories).

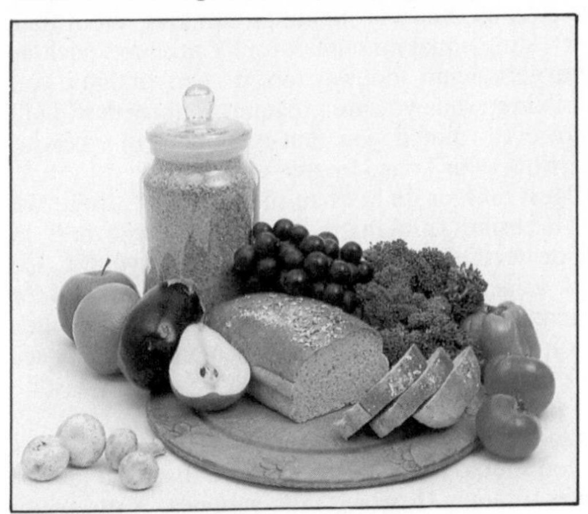

Choose your diet carefully *during pregnancy. Fresh fruit and vegetables, plenty of milk or milk products such as yogurt or cheese, good quantities of protein, and healthy sources of carbohydrate, such as wholemeal bread, are all good news for mothers-to-be.*

Your doctor or midwife will probably also prescribe a prenatal vitamin supplement to help out with two other important items: folacin and iron.

But if you think all this is a lot of eating, consider that if you decide to breast-feed, your eating will have to be even greater than this!

Fluids

While you are pregnant you should drink six to eight glasses of fluid a day, be it water, juice, or milk. This is because your blood volume increases by 25 percent when you are pregnant and your body needs fluid to accomplish that increase.

Fluids are also good for you in several ways: as an aid to digestion (and therefore elimination), as an aid to blood circulation, and as a deterrent to the urinary infections to which pregnant women are more prone.

The downside of all this fluid intake is that you go to the toilet more often, and you are already doing that as the baby grows and seems to jump on your bladder all day and all night.

Calcium

The baby's primary teeth buds form during the fifth month of pregnancy, and the cartilage in the skeleton changes to bone. Calcium is vitally important to your baby's development at all times, but especially during these times.

Your doctor will probably prescribe a prenatal multivitamin which will include calcium, but you should be drinking about four glasses of milk (or eating equal amounts of milk products such as yogurt or cheese) to get calcium that way too. It's a myth that if you don't eat enough calcium while you are pregnant your teeth will fall out. It is true, however, that if you don't get enough calcium, nature will take it from your bones to give to the baby.

If you cannot digest milk or do not like the taste of it, there are other ways to get it besides drinking it. Try cooking with milk in soups or custard desserts. You can also eat cheese, yogurt, ice cream and ice milk to get your milk allotment. (Ice cream and ice milk should be avoided, of course, if you're gaining too much weight. Also be sure to read the ingredients: many types of ice cream and ice milk do not have real milk products in them, despite their name.)

You should not take a calcium supplement without your doctor's permission. And you should not really drink more than four glasses of milk a day since Vitamin D, which milk supplies, is not water

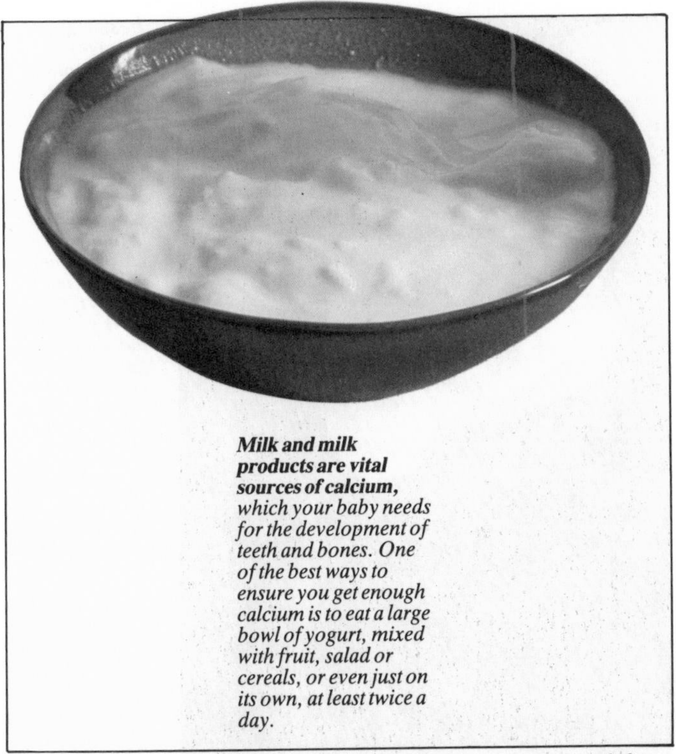

Milk and milk products are vital sources of calcium, *which your baby needs for the development of teeth and bones. One of the best ways to ensure you get enough calcium is to eat a large bowl of yogurt, mixed with fruit, salad or cereals, or even just on its own, at least twice a day.*

soluble. This means that excess amounts are not excreted from your body, which can be bad for you.

SALT

Medical opinion on the benefits or dangers of salt for pregnant women is varied and controversial. Just a few years ago most doctors believed that salt caused toxemia, the swelling of ankles and fingers during pregnancy.

Today, most doctors believe pregnant women need more salt in their diet, not less. This is because your amount of blood and body fluids increases dramatically and you need salt to help retain these fluids. If you don't have this blood and fluid increase it can negatively affect the placenta, and therefore the developing baby. Cutting out salt completely can result in tiredness, irritability, and a loss of appetite.

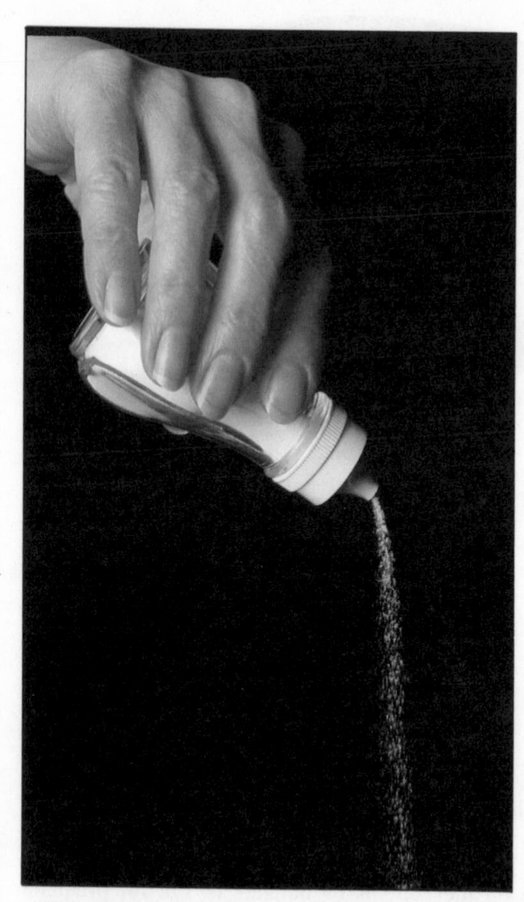

Be sure to get the right amount of salt in your diet. *The best way to judge how much you need is to become aware of your taste buds and to follow their advice — they will tell you clearly if they think you need more salt or less.*

The surest way to determine if you're getting enough salt is the old taste test. Eat whatever amount on your food tastes good, not more. The point is to not eliminate salt from your diet, but just to eat whatever your taste buds tell you.

You should also avoid sea salt in favor of regular table salt with iodine. Iodine is important for normal thyroid functions while you are pregnant.

Of course, don't eat foods with a lot of salt, such as soy sauce, pickles, snack foods (potato chips, for example), and processed meats such as sausage or cured meats.

Cravings

Food cravings are the standard joke about pregnant women. Supposedly you will suddenly develop an urge to have Chinese egg rolls and chocolate-chip ice cream or some such similarly weird combination, at all hours of the day and night.

But food cravings are a myth. The reality is that you may be giving in to a lack of discipline under the guise of "It's because I'm pregnant." You might possibly desire certain foods over others at various times, and these can mean a real dietary need. For example, you may crave salt, but that could be because you need more salt in your diet. Or you may crave vegetables, because you need more vitamins or fiber. If the food you crave is good for you, eat it. But be sensible! This rules out potato chips if you crave salt.

Some women use "food cravings" as a subconscious test of their partner's affection: "If you love me you'll run down to the deli and get me lox and bagels even if it is 4:00 A.M." Don't do this. Talk about it with your partner and explore why you feel this way.

Whatever you think you want to eat, *always try to give your body foods that will do both you and your baby good. Eating at odd times is harmless and may even be something your body needs, but eating odd foods is not.*

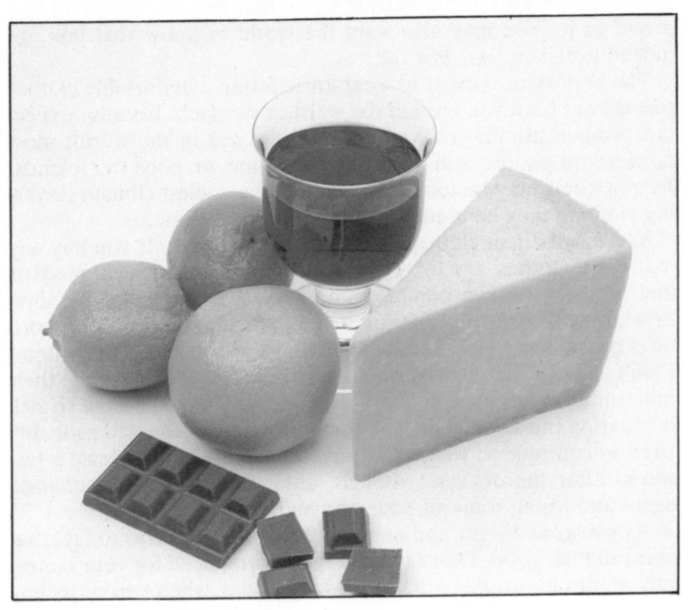

MATERNITY CLOTHING

Maternity clothing has come a long way from the Little Bo-Peep look of just a few years ago. You can still have puffy sleeves and darling little neck-bows if you desire, but you can also have sleek, fashionable outfits that can take you comfortably into the board-room or a night at the opera.

Depending on your pre-pregnant size, you will probably need to go into maternity clothing around the fourth or fifth month. You may not need to wear maternity clothes because you are "showing" but because your regular clothes are uncomfortable.

Incidentally, you may be surprised at the degree to which other people may try to run your life on this point. Some may tell you that you don't "need" to go into maternity clothes yet, that you're not "showing enough." Ignore these people. Only you know how uncomfortable you are in regular clothes. You know how tired you are of safety-pinning your skirts. You can decide to wear maternity clothes any time you want to.

Many women want to get into their maternity clothes as soon as possible, as a sign to the outside world that they are pregnant and proud of it. You may also want the world to know that you are indeed pregnant, not just fat.

The important thing is to wear loose-fitting, comfortable clothes that do not bind you around the waist or stomach. Because expectant women usually feel warmer than the rest of the world, most fabrics you choose will probably be cotton or polyester blends. Heavy wools may be too much, even in the coolest climate (layering clothing may be a good solution in a cold climate).

You may be lent clothes by friends and relatives. If you buy any maternity clothes, try to get mix and match items, such as skirts and blouses you can combine into several outfits. Many a shop assistant will cheerfully tell you that a particular outfit can be worn after pregnancy, just by adding a belt or some such accessory item. Don't believe it: most women say they feel like burning their maternity clothes after delivery, because they have become so sick of wearing the same clothes in the past months. You will probably need to continue to wear your maternity clothes for at least a few weeks after the delivery, though, until you can begin exercising again and losing some of your pregnant weight.

As you grow bigger and more uncomfortable it helps to feel that you still look good. Don't buy everything you need for your maternity wardrobe in one trip. Instead, on a day when you're feeling

Maternity clothing does not have to look drab and shapeless. *Exercise*

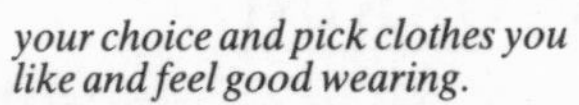

your choice and pick clothes you like and feel good wearing.

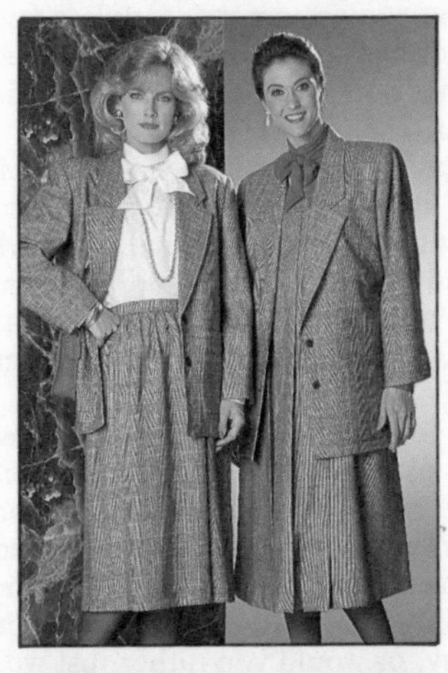

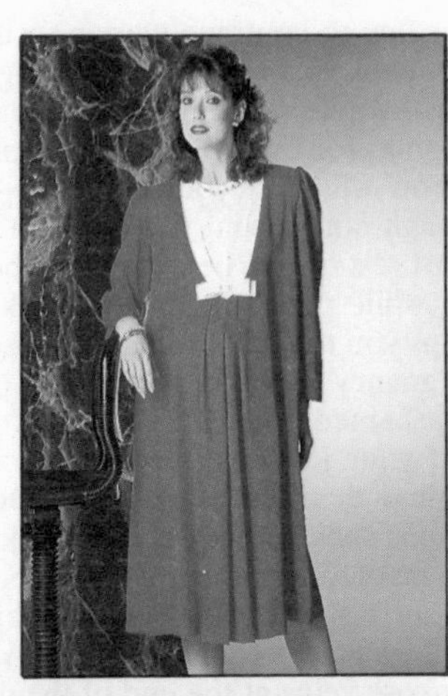

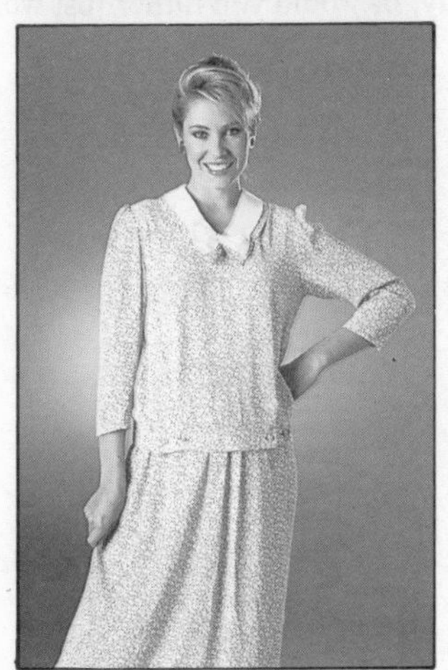

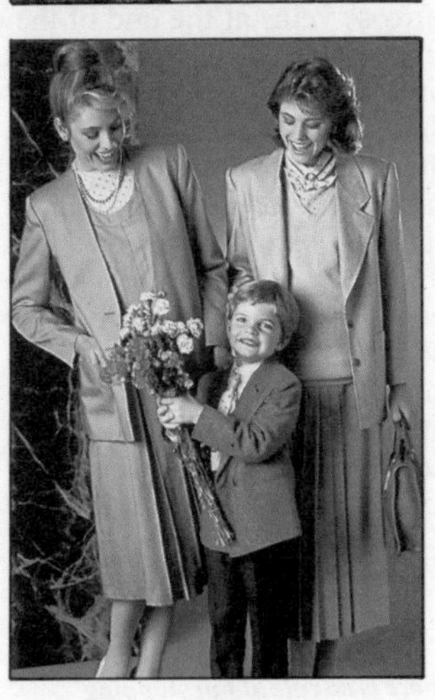

particularly unloved or ugly, it may help to go buy a new sweater or a pretty nursing gown. Of course, it may also help to do anything nice for yourself, such as having a facial or getting your nails done.

WORKING

It is fine to continue working while you are pregnant, unless your job involves a lot of heavy lifting or hard physical labor, or if your job involves working around dangerous chemicals or fumes (including, for example, photographic chemicals).

You will find yourself more easily tired after a day of work though, and again, you shouldn't fight it. Come home and have a short rest or nap before going about your evening activities. Working while pregnant, if you worked before you became pregnant, helps you to feel "normal." It also affirms to the outside world that pregnancy is not an illness, nor is it something to be hidden away, or ashamed about.

If your job involves sitting for long periods, get up and move around as often as possible. Do exercises for individual muscle groups such as neck rolls or ankle rotations while you sit. If your job involves standing, wear support hose and supportive shoes such as nurse's Oxfords. You may have to give up fashionable shoes while you're pregnant. Do you want to have tired, aching feet with varicose veins at the end of the day, or would you rather just wear comfortable if unstylish shoes for a few hours and feel fine? Shift your physical position as often as possible: if sitting, stand up and move around, if standing, sit or lie down.

Use your lunch breaks to rest. Remember that it may take a pregnant woman half a day to recover from extreme fatigue, so don't get worn out! Take it easy, and even baby yourself a little bit. You deserve it.

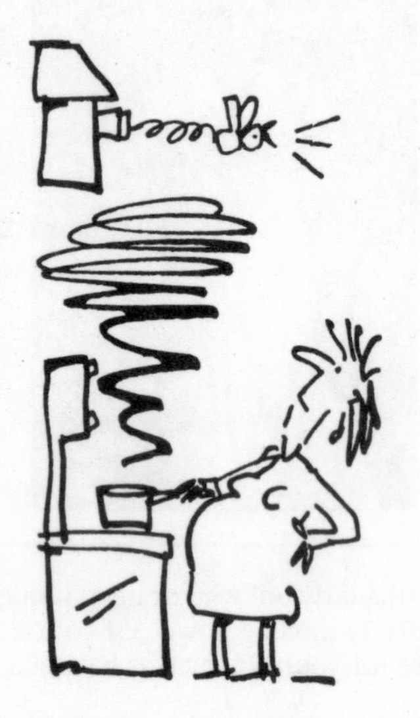

There is no rule about stopping working *when you are pregnant— stop when you feel it's the right time. If you do work, be sure to continue taking all the regular preparatory care of yourself and your child.*

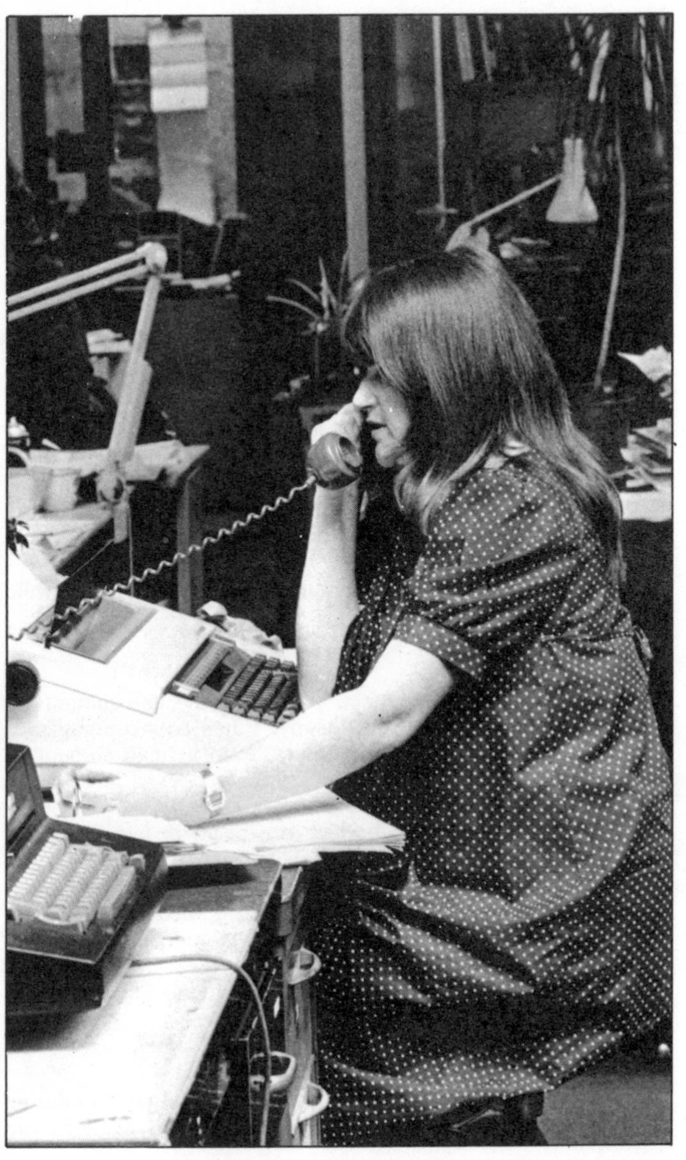

DRUGS AND ALCOHOL

It is not news that drugs are dangerous for you as well as your baby. Some common drugs, such as certain types of antihistamines taken for allergies, can cause permanent birth defects. If a doctor or dentist prescribes medication during pregnancy, get as much information as possible, both about the effect the drug will have on the fetus as well as the effect of not taking the drug at all during your pregnancy. *Make sure your doctor or dentist knows you are pregnant.*

The greatest amount of injury from drugs and medication is during the first trimester (the first three months of pregnancy), when your baby's organs are developing. Talk to your doctor about which common drugs should be avoided (even aspirin has been implicated as a cause of miscarriage).

Street drugs, such as marijuana, heroin, barbiturates, and amphetamines can cause your baby to be born addicted, and means he or she will have to undergo the agony of withdrawal. Street drugs are also considered a possible cause of various malformations and birth defects.

If you love your baby, if not yourself, do not take drugs while you are pregnant.

ALCOHOL

Alcohol is a poison. When taken by an adult in small amounts, it may make us feel relaxed and happy. When passed along to a developing fetus through the placenta, even a small amount of alcohol will make the baby very drunk indeed. And alcohol can damage the baby's developing brain.

"Fetal alcohol syndrome," which can result in facial disfiguration, physical and behavioral problems, heart problems, and mental retardation, is the result of mothers who drink while pregnant, according to the National Institute on Alcohol Abuse and Alcoholism. The Institute recommends no more than two drinks a day.

As with drugs, if you love your growing baby, don't harm it with alcohol.

CAFFEINE

For many women, caffeine is the hardest thing to give up during pregnancy. You can give up alcohol, even cigarettes, but for some

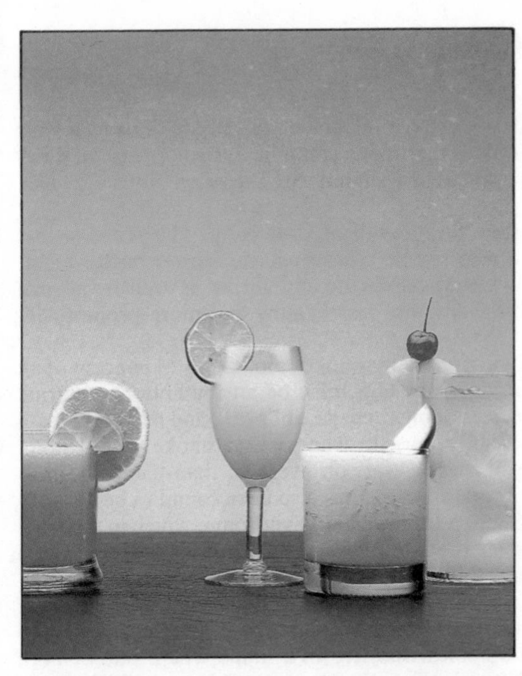

***Attractive cocktails** are just as dangerous for your baby as any other alcoholic drink. Although "safe" levels are recommended, it's best if you can avoid alcohol in any form when you are pregnant.*

reason, that morning cup of coffee is sacred. Part of the problem is that few people realize that caffeine is a drug, but as one doctor eloquently put it: "Would you give your baby narcotics? Then don't consume caffeine."

Easier said than done. But tests done with animals have demonstrated that caffeine can cause stillbirths and miscarriage. This is particularly true when caffeine is not eliminated from the diet during the first three months, when the fetus is first developing.

Doctors recommend that you stop or limit your consumption of caffeine while you are pregnant, especially during the first trimester. Remember that other things besides coffee contain caffeine. A partial list includes: tea, aspirin, cola-flavored soft drinks, even chocolate. Even during the second two trimesters you should seriously try to eliminate or cut down on the amount of caffeine you consume. An upper limit of between four and eight cups a day of a caffeinated item is considered damaging to your baby. Besides, do you feel good when your heart rate is racing and you've got the jitters from caffeine? Neither does your baby!

SMOKING

When you smoke you are cutting down the amount of oxygen your baby receives. And all the toxins you inhale, such as carbon monoxide, lead, and cyanide, are shared with the baby. Not a very nice thought, is it?

These toxins slow the growth of your baby. The result is that babies of women who smoke typically have a lower birth weight. And lower birth-weight babies do not thrive as well as normal birth-weight babies; they are less healthy and more prone to illnesses.

When you smoke, your baby smokes too. Up to 14 per cent of all premature deliveries in the U.S. may be attributable to maternal smoking. The chances of miscarriage, stillbirth, and newborn death become higher. Babies born to women who smoke during pregnancy are seven ounces lighter, on average, than babies born to nonsmokers. Maternal smoking has also been found to be strongly associated with Sudden Infant Death Syndrome, which in the U.S. claims more than six thousand lives a year and is the leading cause of death for children between one and 12 months of age.

If you stop smoking during your pregnancy, stay stopped. Mothers who smoke and breast-feed may be passing nicotine on to their babies. And babies who live in a home where one or both parents smoke have significantly more admissions to the hospital for pneumonia or bronchitis before the age of one year than do infants of nonsmoking parents.

That's a steep price to pay for a habit. But bear in mind that because each cigarette you smoke affects the baby, that means that even reducing the number you smoke will help. Of course, just simply stopping will be even better, but that is admittedly quite difficult for many people.

There are many ways to lower the negative effect of your smoking if you cannot stop altogether.

- Establish no-smoking areas in which you will *not* light up a cigarette; for example, the car, your office, your kitchen. The more areas you make off-limits

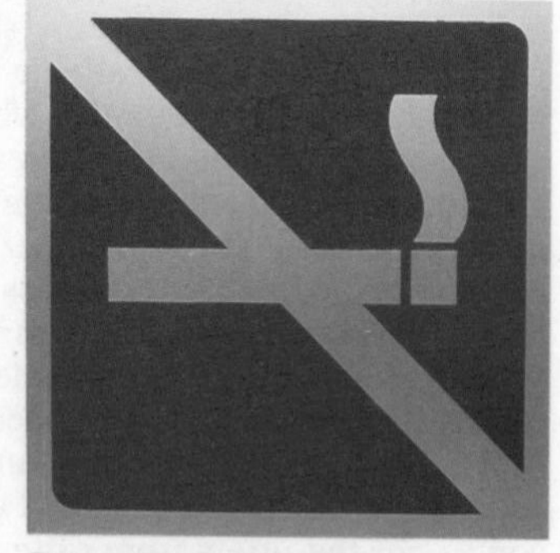

Put up "No Smoking" signs.

to smoking, the more you will cut down the opportunities you have for smoking.

- Establish no-smoking activities. For example, you can arbitrarily say you won't smoke while listening to music, while reading a book, while talking on the telephone, while ironing. This will also have the effect of cutting down your opportunities for smoking.
- Switch to a low-tar or low-nicotine brand.
- Don't buy cigarettes in cartons; buy one pack at a time. You may get tired of having to run to the store every time you need another pack, which will also cut down your smoking.
- Don't inhale so deeply.
- Put out your cigarette halfway, or even better, after two puffs.
- Store your cigarette pack somewhere that is difficult to get to, or is troublesome to find.
- Stay away from other smokers and out of smoke-filled rooms. You and your baby still receive the negative effects of cigarette smoke from these secondary sources, even if you are not smoking.

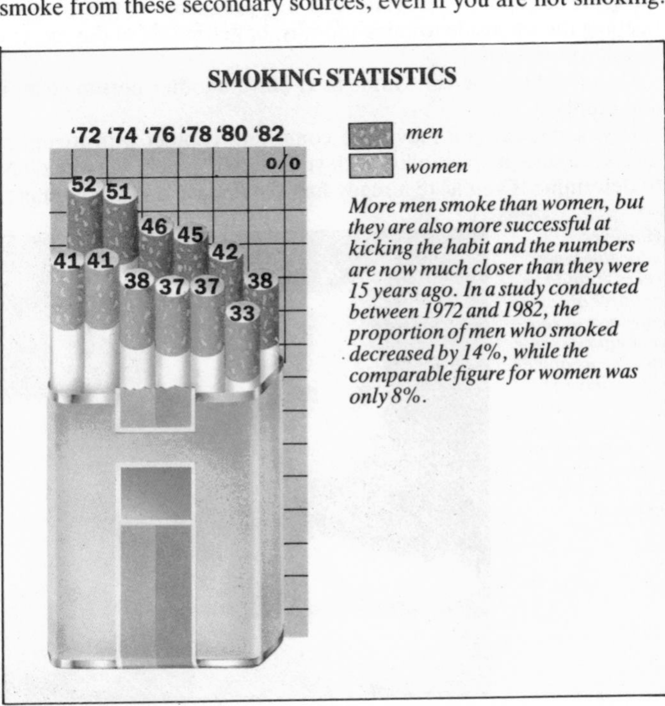

SMOKING STATISTICS

More men smoke than women, but they are also more successful at kicking the habit and the numbers are now much closer than they were 15 years ago. In a study conducted between 1972 and 1982, the proportion of men who smoked decreased by 14%, while the comparable figure for women was only 8%.

CATS

As much as you may love your cat, beware of it during pregnancy; cats can carry a disease, toxoplasmosis, that is potentially life-threatening to the fetus. Toxoplasmosis is caused by eating raw meat or by coming into contact with an animal, usually a cat, that has eaten raw meat and is a carrier of the disease.

Toxoplasmosis can cause retardation, blindness, or fatal illness in the developing baby. Chances of infection are highest in the final three months of pregnancy when the disease can also cause the most neurological problems.

Do not eat raw or undercooked meat (this includes sushi, or raw fish Japanese-style, unfortunately). Don't feed raw or undercooked meat to your cat. Instead give it only canned or dry food, or cooked meat. Stop your cat, if you can, from hunting and eating mice, birds, and so on while you are pregnant. If this involves keeping the cat inside for nine months, or getting rid of the cat, you should consider it.

Do not touch the cat's litter box. Have another person clean it and empty it.

If you suspect you may have come into contact with toxoplasmosis, discuss the possibility with your doctor. There is a blood test to determine if you have already had the disease and are immune.

However adorable your cat is, *it could be a source of infection to you and your newborn baby. Try to have a friend care for the cat while you are pregnant, or have someone else look after it at home.*

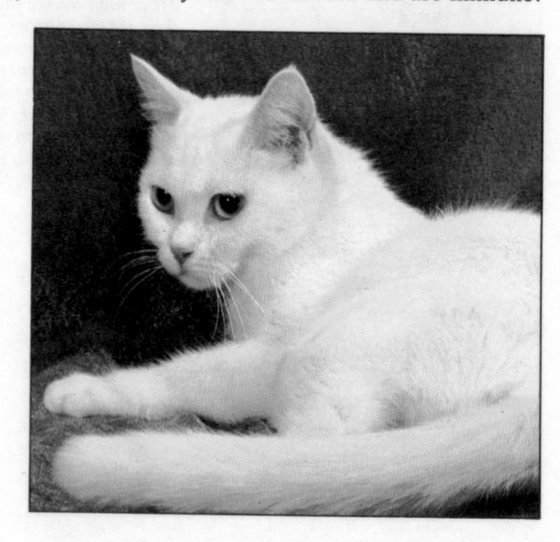

TRAVELING

It is usually perfectly all right to travel while you are pregnant, provided you have your doctor's permission for long trips. But you should exercise some common sense when traveling.

Long trips by plane or car will be especially tiring when you are pregnant. Do not stay seated longer than two hours—you should get up and move around more often if you can.

From about the seventh month until you deliver, it's probably wise to stay closer to home, primarily because babies, especially first babies, are unpredictable in when they choose to arrive. There is very little danger that you'll deliver on the way to a hospital, but do you want to deliver your baby in a strange city with a doctor you haven't met before?

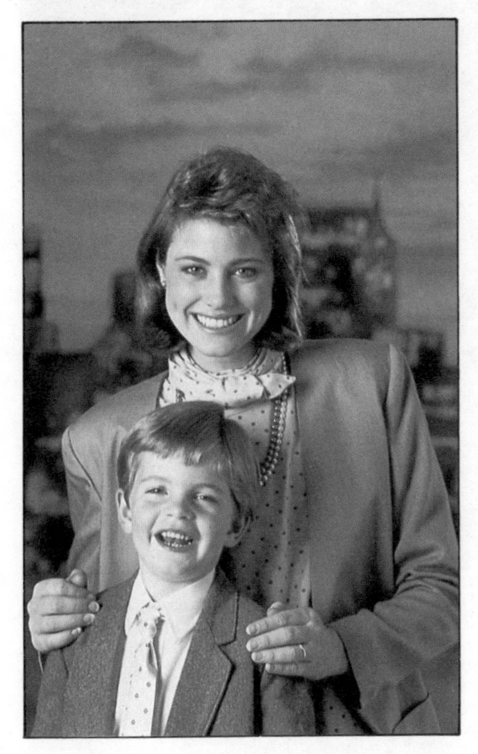

When you are pregnant there is nothing to stop you traveling *if you want to, but remember that there are two of you to look after. Take a bit more care than you might normally do, and expect to find yourself more easily tired than usual. It's also a good time to travel with your other children, if this is something you enjoy.*

SEX

Sex got you to this point in life, yet sex can be a very touchy subject during pregnancy. Basically, it's OK to have a sexual relationship with your partner while you are pregnant; in fact, now is a time when your sexual relationship may become even more fulfilling.

Particularly during the first six months, sex is perfectly safe and requires no change from your usual practices. As you enter the last three months, your increasing size may make some positions awkward or uncomfortable—you may have to make some adjustments. Many doctors suggest that you avoid intercourse during the last four weeks of your pregnancy, since there is a chance it will cause premature labor.

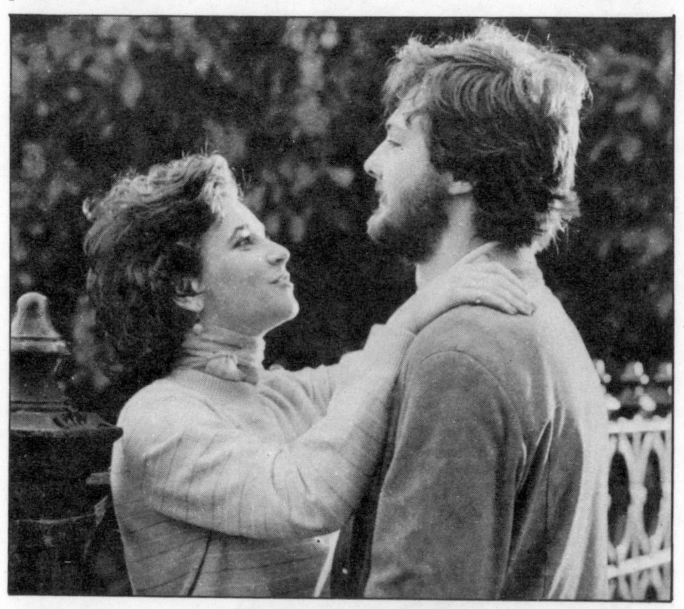

***Your own self-image** and your partner's image of you will change continually during your pregnancy, but need not affect your sex life for the first six months. In the later stages of pregnancy as the baby grows larger, discuss the most comfortable position with your partner. Consult your doctor if you have any worries at all.*

Be aware that there may be lots of conflicting feelings and emotions while you are pregnant. One or both of you may be afraid to have sex. Try to be open and communicate about it. A number of factors come into play: fear of hurting the baby is the most dominant. Conventional sexual intercourse cannot infect or harm the baby—it is safely protected inside a closed cervix and cushioned by the amniotic sac.

Another big stumbling block to full enjoyment of sex during pregnancy is negative body image. You may feel disgusted with your blossoming figure, your stretch marks, and the new odors and excretions of your pregnant body. Or your partner may feel this way. To really complicate things, you can use double-think and project your feelings of disgust with your own body onto your partner and convince yourself that surely he is repelled by your fatness, when in truth your partner is probably delighted by your shape and finds you beautiful and radiant!

Another disconcerting factor: the baby's reaction to your lovemaking may be an increase in its activity. Don't worry: your baby isn't watching!

There are some cautions to having sex during pregnancy, though. Bleeding or pain during intercourse should be reported to your doctor. Your partner's full weight should not be placed upon your stomach—this is uncomfortable for you as well as the baby. This is a time to try new positions other than the conventional "missionary" position.

If you have any doubts or hesitation about sex during pregnancy, discuss them fully with your doctor or midwife.

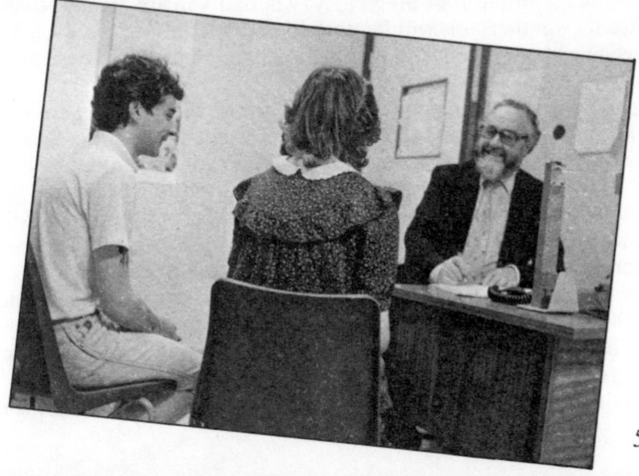

EMOTIONS

Pregnant women are a hotbed of emotions. The hormonal changes that run rampant through your body cause an increase in emotional response. Whatever your feelings, they are yours and they are real, regardless of how ridiculous they might sound.

Pregnant women's emotions run the gamut from wonder, delight, and joy to raging frustration, fear and depression. Unexplained outbursts, crying, and anxiety are not unusual—all in a matter of hours. This aspect of pregnancy is perhaps most bewildering to your partner, who must stand by helplessly. Your mind and your body are experiencing major changes to the extent that it can be considered a life crisis, since your entire lifestyle and self-identity are being dramatically changed.

Talk to someone about all your emotions and fears. Whether that someone be your partner, a relative, or a friend, talk, talk, talk. The only rule for your listening post is that he or she should not argue with you—there is no right or wrong to emotions, there just *is* emotion.

You may feel frightened, ambivalent, or full of anticipatory joy about the coming birth. You may also feel all three of these emotions almost simultaneously. It's normal, it's typical, it's fine to feel this way. You're OK.

It is a myth that a pregnant woman should walk around blissfully happy for nine months, radiant in the certain knowledge that she will soon be a mommy and fulfilled, etc., etc. You may well feel conflict regarding your pregnancy: whether you are "ready" to be a parent, whether you will be able to care for, afford, or even love this new little person who is going to disrupt your life. These are all normal fears.

It is important to come to terms with the fact that you are pregnant and you will be a mommy. Many women ignore the fact that they are pregnant for at least the first few months, until they begin to show and feel more pregnant. You will no longer be just you, you will have the care and feeding of another person in your life. And while there is a great deal of joy in caring for another person, there is also a lot of work and sleepless nights. You will be a parent, not just a mommy of a cute little baby, and parents have to deal with rebellious children and difficult decisions.

Talk to your partner about your emotions and your fears. Talk to yourself about it too, by keeping a journal.

Understand that your partner may also be going through some

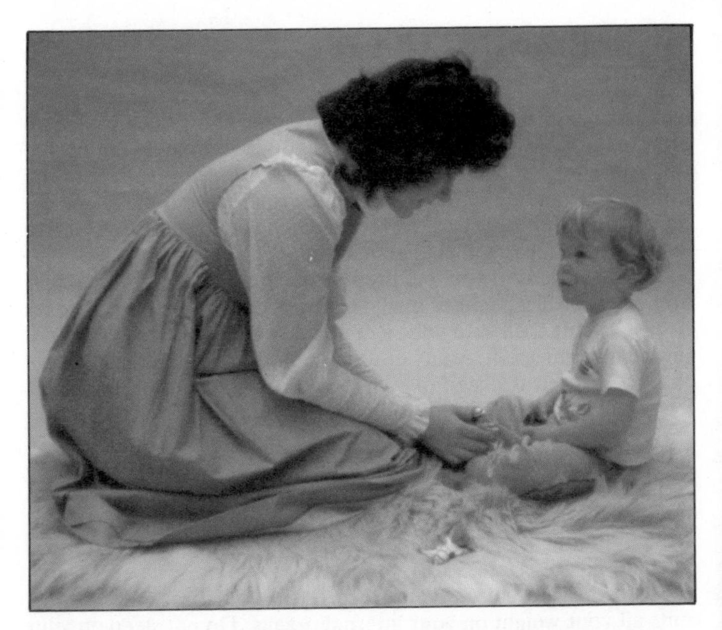

***Pregnancy is a very emotional time,** not only for you but also for other members of your family. Sharing your own feelings and theirs is for many people the best way to ensure a happy pregnancy.*

emotional changes. He is about to be a father, and that can be frightening and stressful, too. He may fear that he is unable to take care of you and the baby adequately, with the result that he works longer and harder to earn more money. He may also fear losing his independence, as well as losing the independent woman who suddenly seems to need him more. He may fear the intrusion of a third person into your cozy twosome. He may be jealous of the baby's importance and closeness to you, or your closeness to other nurturing people such as your mother or sister, during your pregnancy.

Many men also feel jealous that they cannot procreate in the same way women do. These men can be almost obsessively concerned with everything to do with pregnancy and may counter their feelings by working harder at their jobs, or taking on new jobs, or more creative jobs. Some expectant fathers exhibit the symptoms of pregnancy; fatigue, dizziness, heartburn, weight gain. This is a time of great emotional change for your partner, too, and you should be aware of and understanding of that fact.

SLEEP AND DREAMS

You'll experience a major increase in your need for sleep while you are pregnant. Many women report that this is greatest during the first trimester; others say that they require more sleep at about the fifth or sixth month; still others say the final three months are the most tiring. Suffice it to say every woman is different. But fatigue and sleep patterns will change markedly.

The first rule is: if you feel tired, rest. Your body is working hard and you need sleep and/or rest. That need may be for several hours or just a short spell with your feet up and your eyes closed (and the phone disconnected). Many of today's hard-driving women believe that to be tired is a sign of weakness or a "womanly complaint." They will fight the feeling of fatigue, ignoring their need to sleep or rest. Such women need to acknowledge that pregnancy is a time of great physical work on the part of their body, and they *need* rest.

This isn't to say you should walk around feeling like a wet noodle. Excessive fatigue should be reported to your doctor. Pregnancy, although a time of major changes in your body, is also a normal, healthy state.

Sleep on your side. Avoid sleeping on your back because this puts all your weight on your internal organs. Do not sleep on your stomach, for obvious reasons (it will also be uncomfortable, because of your growing breasts and your growing tummy).

If you cannot comfortably share a bed with your partner—this will probably happen during the final months of your pregnancy—sleep apart from him so both of you can get a decent night's rest. You're going to need all the sleep you can get before the baby arrives.

You will also notice that you probably have to get up several times in the night to urinate. Try not drinking anything for about an hour or so before bedtime (and bedtime, by the way, should be early when you're pregnant). If you still find yourself trudging wearily to the bathroom in the middle of the night, think of it as good practice for waking up when your newborn cries.

Dreams

Dreams and nightmares seem especially vivid while you are pregnant; they can be truly frightening. For some reason, dreams seem more real when you're pregnant. Discuss them with your partner and treat them as ways to understand yourself and this strange process called pregnancy. But don't make the disturbing mistake of thinking your dreams or nightmares signal reality. They are only dreams.

Most dreams center on the baby in some way. These commonly have themes of somehow mistreating the baby—not caring for it properly, hurting it by, for example, not feeding it, or even forgetting where you put the baby. You may even dream that the baby is dead, or shrivelled up. Before you wake up the neighborhood, remember that this is a dream and probably signals only your concern that the baby will be ill or die, not that there is already something wrong with the baby in your uterus.

Other dreams typically concern you and your partner, and how your relationship relates to the baby. Usually these dreams involve abandonment by your partner of you and the baby. It doesn't mean it's going to happen, it means you are aware of how vulnerable you and a newborn will be. Talk to your partner about this, express your need for reassurance, and *accept* the reassurances. Remember that he too is probably feeling some of the same fears you are experiencing.

On the other hand, you may also have unusually pleasant dreams about enjoying your baby. Many women report dreaming more than once that they have given birth after an almost painless labor and delivery.

Insomnia

Some women have trouble getting to sleep or staying asleep during pregnancy. Often this is caused simply because you are physically uncomfortable—the need to urinate more often, the baby's kicking, heartburn, and your increasing size late in pregnancy can make it difficult to sleep. Late at night is also often the time for worrying —a great way to keep yourself awake.

You need your rest, so try doing some relaxation exercises before going to sleep. (You will learn these techniques in your exercise and childbirth classes.) If this doesn't help, admit that you can't sleep. Don't stay in bed, tossing and turning (and keeping your partner awake); get up and do something constructive, and try to catch up on your sleep later.

Whatever steps you take to deal with insomnia, *don't* take any sort of drug. It is far better to feel sleepy than to risk damaging your unborn child.

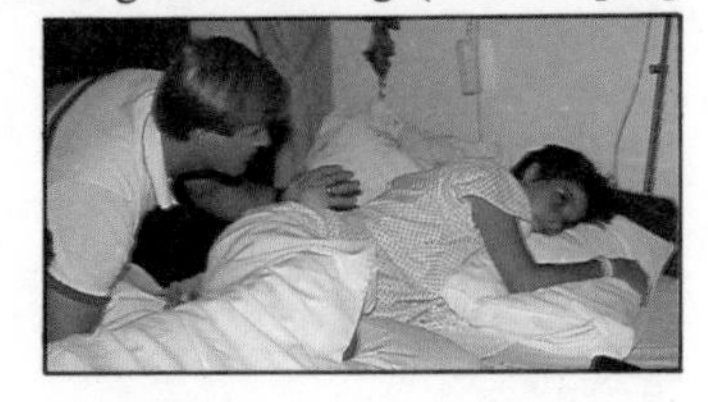

Your partner can be a great help.

NAMING YOUR BABY

It takes some people weeks to name a kitten or puppy, so it's best to start thinking about baby names early in your pregnancy. You will find you receive all kinds of uninvited "help" with this process, from relatives as well as well-meaning friends. This is *your* baby and *you* get to choose the name. In fact, in most states only the mother signs the birth certificate, so ultimately it is up to you alone.

One method of deciding your child's name is for you and your partner to write down several names for both girls and boys that you each like. Any names that occur on both lists are good candidates for baby names.

Of course, you'll want to consider any traditional family names. On the other hand, you may want to choose a distinctive, unusual name. Whatever you decide, think about your child when you choose its name. If you really want to call your pride and joy Moondrop Chastity, think of what that child will endure at school from teachers and schoolmates (and remember that young children are quite often unkind to each other). Think too about what the child's initials spell, and any nicknames that could be derived from either the name or the initials with which your child could be teased.

It's also probably a good idea to keep whatever names you decide upon, or are seriously considering, to yourselves. People will ask what names you've picked and when you tell them, jaws will drop, eyebrows will arch, and you will get their uninvited opinion of the name you have chosen. If the opinion is negative, it can be disturbing and unduly influence your choice. It can also be hurtful if the name you have chosen has special sentimental meaning for you and your partner.

Keep a running list of your current top contenders. You may be amazed and amused to find how different they are from the name you finally select.

THE MOST POPULAR GIRLS' NAMES

Adrienne
Alicia
Alison
Allison
Amanda
Amber
Amy
Andrea
Angela
Anna
Anne
Ann
April
Ashley
Audrey
Beth
Bethany
Bonnie
Brandy
Bridget
Brittany
Brooke
Caitlin
Candice
Caroline
Carolyn
Carrie
Catherine
Chelsea
Christina
Christine
Courtney
Crystal
Dana
Danielle
Dawn
Ellen
Elizabeth
Emily
Erica
Erika
Erin
Gina
Hannah
Heather
Heidi
Holly
Jacqueline
Jaime
Jamie
Jean
Jennifer
Jessica
Jillian
Jodi
Julia
Julie
Karen
Kari
Kate
Katherine
Kathryn
Kathleen
Katie
Katy
Kayla
Kelly
Kimberly
Kirsten
Kristen
Kristin
Kristina
Laura
Lauren
Leah
Leslie
Lindsay
Lindsey
Lisa
Maria
Marie
Marissa
Mary
Megan
Meghan
Melanie
Melinda
Melissa
Michele
Michelle
Molly
Natalie
Nichole
Nicole
Pamela
Rachel
Rebecca
Renee
Samantha
Sara
Sarah
Shanna
Shannon
Sheena
Stacey
Stacy
Stephanie
Susan
Tamara
Tara
Theresa
Tiffany
Tina
Valarie
Valerie
Vanessa
Veronica
Victoria

THE MOST POPULAR BOYS' NAMES

Aaron
Adam
Alan
Alexander
Allen
Andrew
Andy
Anthony
Benjamin
Blake
Bobby
Brad
Bradley
Brandon
Brent
Brett
Brian
Bryan
Carl
Chad
Charles
Chase
Christian
Christopher
Cody
Colin
Cory
Craig
Curtis
Dane
Daniel
Danny
Darren
David
Derek
Donald
Douglas
Drew
Dustin
Edward
Evan
Eric
Erik
Frank
Gabriel
Gary
Geoffrey
George
Grant
Gregory
Ian
Jacob
James
Jamie
Jared
Jason
Jeffrey
Jeremy
Jesse
Joel
John
Jonathan
Jordan
Joseph
Joshua
Justin
Keith
Kenneth
Kevin
Kyle
Lawrence
Louis
Luke
Marcus
Mark
Matthew
Michael
Nathan
Nathaniel
Nicholas
Patrick
Paul
Peter
Philip
Phillip
Richard
Robert
Russell
Ryan
Samuel
Scott
Sean
Seth
Shane
Shaun
Shawn
Stephen
Steven
Taylor
Thomas
Timothy
Todd
Travis
Trevor
Tyler
William
Vincent
Zachary

SUPPLIES FOR THE BABY

The most basic thing a baby needs is *you* and the nurturing and warmth you provide. But there are many other things your infant will require. It's a good idea to acquire these before you go to the hospital. Here are a few essentials to start off with:

FURNITURE

You may already have furniture for the nursery, or you may be given or lent furniture. In that case, or if you are buying new, be sure everything is in good condition and meets federal safety standards. You'll need:

- crib or bassinet—remember, babies outgrow bassinets very quickly
- changing table with safety strap
- dresser or bureau for clothing and supplies
- comfortable rocking chair for nursing and soothing your baby

INFANT CAR SEAT

Some states, such as California, require that your baby be in a suitable car seat; the hospital may not release your baby to you unless you have one to take the baby home. Babies should *never* be removed from their car seats while the car is moving. If you have to feed or change the baby, pull over and take a rest stop. Your doctor or clinic can give you recommendations as to which brands are considered safe.

INFANT SEAT

This is useful for placing the baby in an upright position for feeding or just so that it can watch you. Be sure that the seat has a safety strap.

STROLLER

This should be stable with a brake and a safe mechanism for collapsing the stroller. Anticipate where your baby's fingers and toes could get stuck or pinched and avoid strollers that have these traps. The best idea is to test the stroller with your baby in it.

CLOTHING

Babies need clean clothing with remarkable frequency. The more you have to begin with, the less time you will spend doing laundry:

● cloth diapers—at least a dozen even if you use disposable diapers, five or six dozen if you don't ● six receiving blankets ● ten cotton undershirts ● three caps ● four terry stretch jump-suits ● six cotton nightgowns ● one snowsuit ● two or three sweaters

SUPPLIES

A happy baby needs love and also:
● three crib sheets ● rubberized flannel sheet ● six soft wash-cloths and towels ● diaper rash ointment ● cotton balls ● cotton swabs ● soft hairbrush ● rectal thermometer ● petroleum jelly ● safety pins if you use cloth diapers ● bottles, nipples, and sterilizer if you bottle-feed ● two eight-ounce and two four-ounce bottles with nipples if you breast-feed

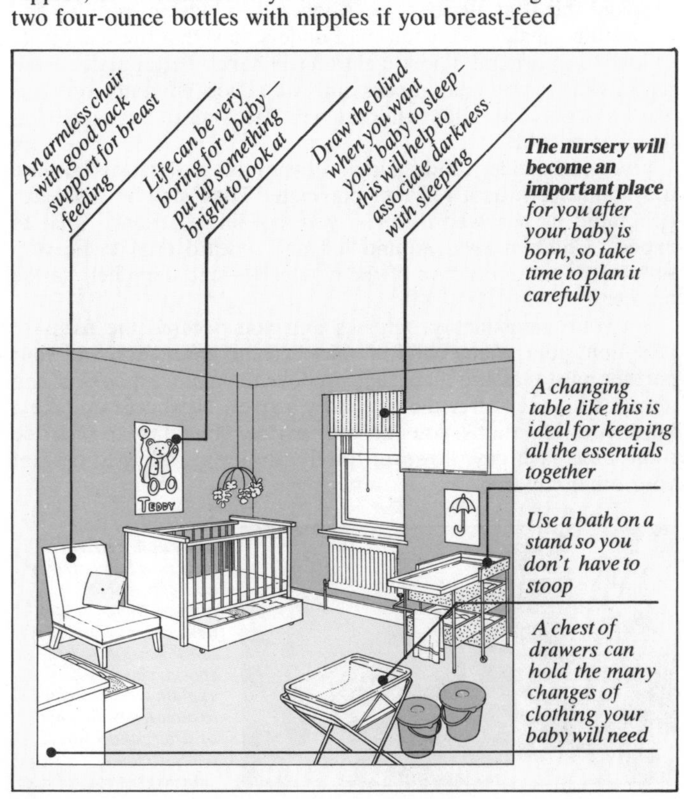

An armless chair with good back support for breast feeding
Life can be very boring for a baby—put up something bright to look at
Draw the blind when you want your baby to sleep—this will help to associate darkness with sleeping
TEDDY
A changing table like this is ideal for keeping all the essentials together
Use a bath on a stand so you don't have to stoop
A chest of drawers can hold the many changes of clothing your baby will need

The nursery will become an important place *for you after your baby is born, so take time to plan it carefully*

SIBLINGS

You should begin preparing your other child (or children) for the arrival of a little brother or sister as early as possible. It is best to do this as gently and as lovingly as possible, particularly if the child has been an only child so far.

Toddlers often have the hardest time adjusting to a new baby, since they perceive the new arrival as taking their place. Talk to toddlers a lot about the coming baby. Let them feel the baby move in your belly, and explain that a new baby is growing in a special place inside you. You may upset a toddler if you move him or her from his current sleeping place to make room for the new baby; try to avoid this if at all possible. Above all, be loving, positive and reassuring—make sure your child understands that there is plenty of love to go around. Older children will have a better understanding of what a new baby means and will almost certainly look forward to its arrival. Older children will also want to be involved as much as possible.

One reason older children look forward to a new baby is because they think of it as a resident playmate. They may be sadly disappointed by a newborn unless you explain in advance what to expect. Children aged around ten and upward tend to be very supportive and protective of the new baby—and a big help to the mother.

As your pregnancy progresses and you become the focus of attention, your young children may become upset. You and your partner must reassure them that you love them more than ever and always will, even after the new baby arrives. Newborns do take a lot of your attention—you and your partner should try to set aside some time each day, however briefly, to devote solely to each of your other children.

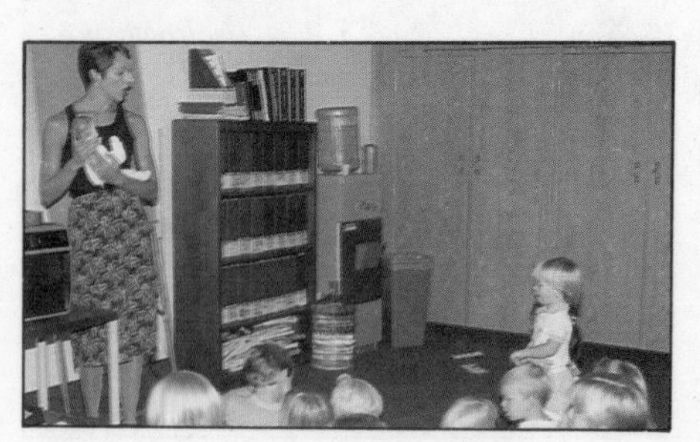

Don't forget your other children *when your new baby arrives and, if possible, prepare them for the newcomer in advance. Some schools offer special classes to explain what it means to have a new brother or sister, and your pediatrician will also be able to give you advice.*

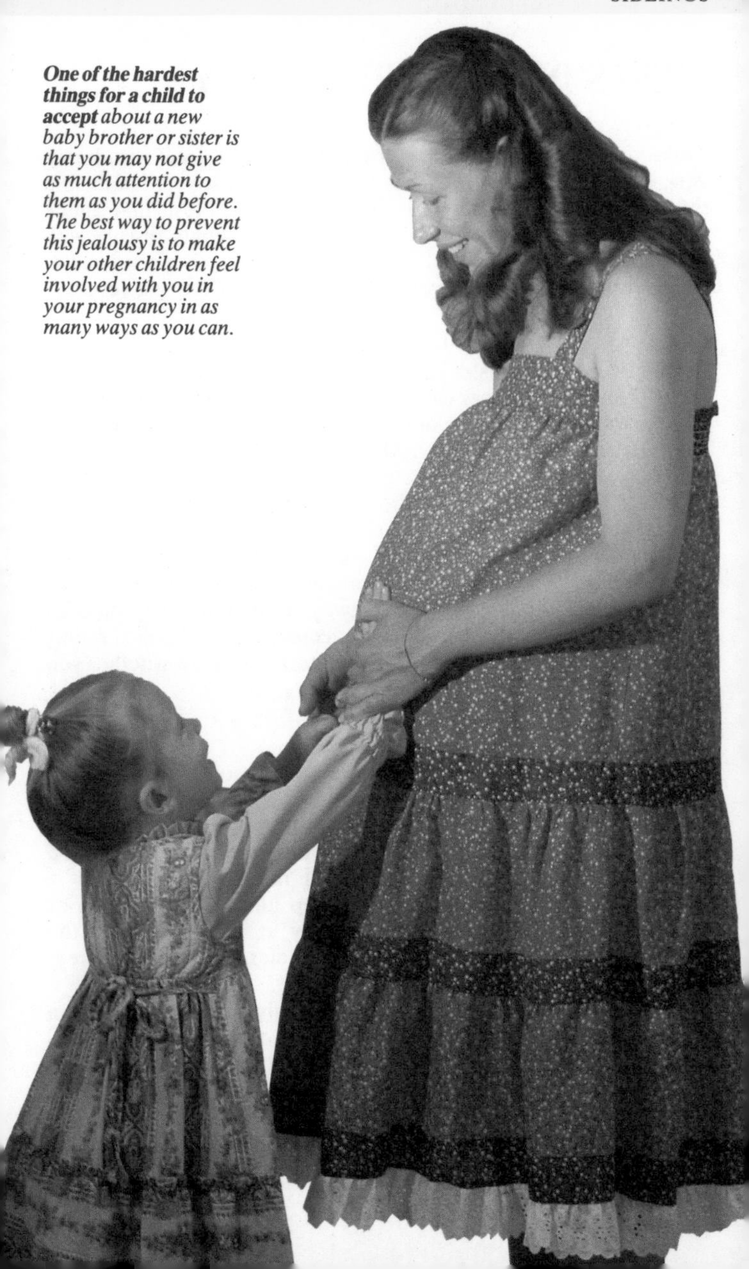

***One of the hardest things for a child to accept** about a new baby brother or sister is that you may not give as much attention to them as you did before. The best way to prevent this jealousy is to make your other children feel involved with you in your pregnancy in as many ways as you can.*

TESTS DURING PREGNANCY

There are several standard tests that your doctor will run during various stages of your pregnancy to determine that your health and the baby's are good. There are also some optional tests that can be given, depending on a variety of factors. You should discuss with your doctor or midwife what each test is for, how it is given, what it will determine, and when you will be notified of the test results.

GERMAN MEASLES (RUBELLA)

Because German measles can cause serious problems in the developing fetus if the mother catches it, a standard blood test to determine immunity to this type of measles is almost always given during the early stages of pregnancy. Ideally, you should be tested before you become pregnant: if you are not immune then you will be vaccinated, which means you should not then become pregnant for at least three months.

If you accidentally come into contact with someone who has German measles while you are pregnant (children other than your own are good candidates to stay away from, since they pick up childhood diseases through day-care centers and schools), report this to your doctor immediately. Blood tests will show whether you have been infected.

RHESUS STATUS

After a baby is born or after a miscarriage, some of the baby's blood enters the mother's circulatory system. In some cases, the mother's Rhesus blood group is Rh-positive, while the baby's is Rh-negative. This difference, called Rh incompatibility, causes the mother to develop antibodies against Rh-negative blood.

Since antibodies almost never develop until after the birth or miscarriage, first babies are very rarely at risk. However, the mother continues to produce the antibodies. In her next pregnancy, the antibodies could harm the fetus.

Fortunately, a vaccination can now be given to women after a birth or miscarriage to destroy any blood cells that may have entered the mother's system and to prevent the antibodies from forming. This has reduced the problem of Rh incompatibility considerably.

At the beginning of your pregnancy you will be given a blood test to see if your blood is Rh-positive or Rh-negative. If you are Rh-negative, then the father's blood should also be tested. If there is a chance that the baby will have Rh-positive blood, you will need to have regular blood tests throughout your pregnancy, even if it is your first.

HEMOGLOBIN LEVEL

If the hemoglobin in your red blood cells falls below a certain level, you are anemic and your cells will not get enough oxygen. The symptoms of mild anemia are not really noticeable, but in more severe cases you may be short of breath, and be pale, weak, and tired. You may even faint or have heart palpitations.

Anemia during pregnancy usually is caused by too little iron or too little folic acid (Vitamin B6) in your body. This could be because you are not eating properly, or it could be that the changes in your body are affecting your ability to absorb these nutrients from your food. Be sure to eat properly and include lots of green, leafy vegetables in your diet. Your doctor will probably prescribe iron and folic acid supplements even if you are not anemic.

BLOOD TESTS FOR GENETIC DISEASES

Certain ethnic groups are prone to some genetically linked diseases. If both the father and mother are carriers of a disease (even though they show no signs of having it), it could be passed on to the unborn child. If you fall into a high-risk category, you should discuss the possibilities with your doctor and have the appropriate blood tests; if you carry the genetic trait, the baby's father should be tested as well. People of black African origin are prone to sickle-cell anemia; people of Mediterranean, Middle Eastern, and Far Eastern origin are prone to another form of anemia called thalassemia. People of Eastern European Jewish descent should be tested for Tay-Sachs and related diseases.

VENEREAL DISEASE

Some doctors and clinics routinely run blood tests for venereal disease. The most common venereal disease today is herpes simplex type II, and it is therefore not considered an unusual complication of pregnancy. If you have this virus you will be tested at certain points throughout your pregnancy for any signs of outbreak of the disease. If a woman has an outbreak at the time of delivery it is almost always necessary to deliver by Caesarean section for the baby's health: a baby passing through an infected birth canal or cervix can be jeopardized.

Alpha Fetoprotein Testing

This blood test is intended to determine whether the fetus is suffering from any one of several abnormalities of the central nervous system, such as spina bifida, or Down's syndrome. Some states, such as California, strongly recommend the test be administered, but it is still the mother's choice. It is administered at 16 weeks of pregnancy. Unusually high results are typically followed by an ultrasound scan or amniocentesis to see if the fetal head or spinal column are showing signs of any of the diseases.

Urine Tests

Generally, you will be asked to bring in a urine sample to every doctor visit. These should be early-morning specimens, since urine is more concentrated at that time.

The presence of protein in your urine warns of a urinary tract infection in early pregnancy, or the possible development of toxemia in later pregnancy.

The presence of sugar in your urine is a possible indication of diabetes. It is not unusual to have sugar in your urine sometimes, but the sugar level stays consistently high, you will be tested for diabetes.

If either of these illnesses show up, appropriate treatment can be given.

Ultrasound

Ultrasound scans—which have no effect on the fetus or the mother—are used for a variety of reasons, including: to determine the stage of the pregnancy, to detect twins, to show the baby's growth, and to see the baby's position in the womb.

Ultrasound is a simple and painless procedure. The ultrasound device sends sound waves through your body tissues and records their echoes as they encounter the fetus. The sound waves are translated into an image on a monitor screen and can also be made into a photograph.

There are no known drawbacks to ultrasound. The fetus may react to the high-frequency sound the test sends through your womb with an increase in its activity.

You will be asked to drink four to five tall glasses of water about an hour before the test and then hold them in. This, as your pregnancy advances, is an exceedingly difficult and uncomfortable thing to do. The fluid is necessary for the sound waves to pass through your womb and give a picture of the baby. If you become especially uncomfortable (and your kidneys will cry out for mercy after about

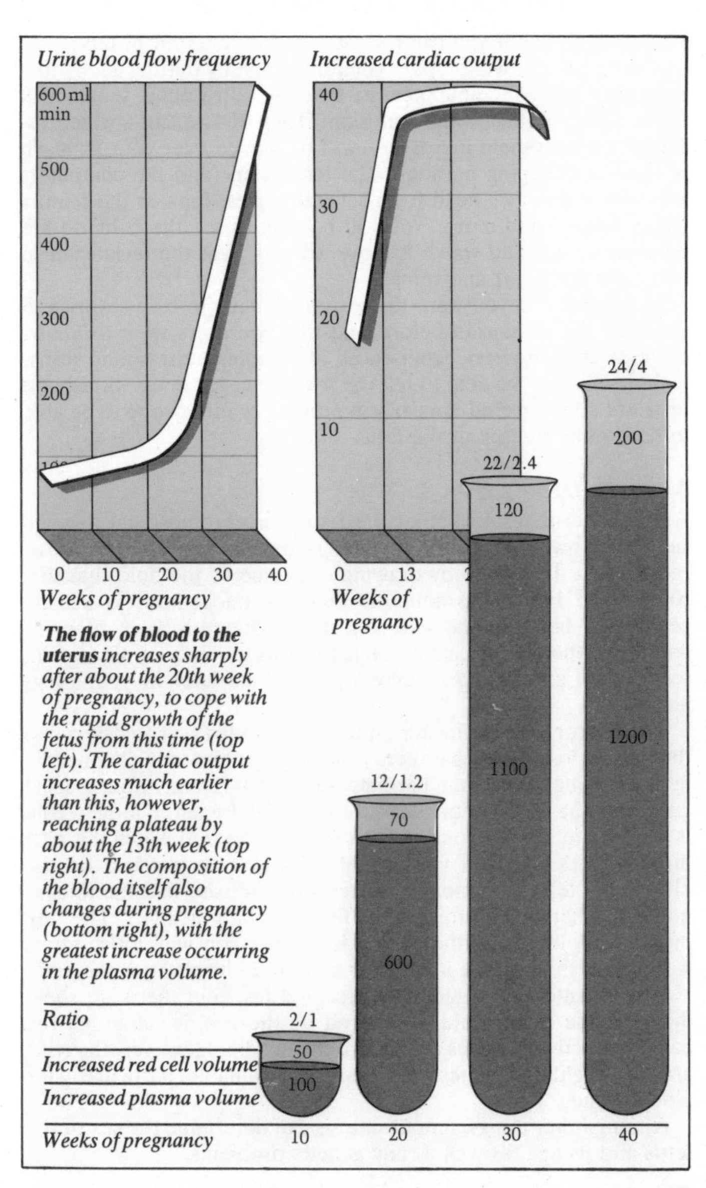

***The flow of blood to the uterus** increases sharply after about the 20th week of pregnancy, to cope with the rapid growth of the fetus from this time (top left). The cardiac output increases much earlier than this, however, reaching a plateau by about the 13th week (top right). The composition of the blood itself also changes during pregnancy (bottom right), with the greatest increase occurring in the plasma volume.*

90 minutes), ask if you can release a certain amount of fluid.

The technician will prepare you for the test by putting a jelly-like substance on your abdomen so that the ultrasound sensor will make solid contact with your skin. Then the sensor—which resembles a hand-held hairdryer—will be moved over your stomach in several sweeping motions. The technician (and the computer) measure the baby's head from several angles, look at the femurs (thigh bones) and more. You will be able to see the baby on the monitor screen and watch it move around. Ask the technician to point out the heart and spine.

Incidentally, if you want the sex of the baby to be a surprise to you, tell the technician beforehand that you don't want to know. Because they are very experienced at "reading" ultrasound scans, technicians may be able to tell the sex. However, most ultrasound tests are administered too early in pregnancy for anyone to be able to determine the sex of the fetus.

Amniocentesis

Amniocentesis tests whether the fetus has chromosomal damage such as Down's syndrome, which results in various degrees of retardation. It is done by drawing out some of the fluid that surrounds the baby—the amniotic fluid. Amniocentesis is usually performed between the sixteenth and eighteenth week of pregnancy. If there is a chance of a premature birth or Caesarean section, an amniocentesis may also be done later in your pregnancy.

The doctor will administer an ultrasound scan first to determine the baby's position so that there is no danger of inserting the needle in the wrong place and harming the fetus. Then, after a local anesthetic has been administered to your abdomen, a long needle is inserted into your stomach (you may not want to watch this part directly, although you will probably be able to watch it on the ultrasound television monitor to reassure yourself that the fetus is not being harmed by this rather fierce-looking needle). The tiny puncture hole left by the needle is all that you will notice afterward. You should take it easy for at least 24 hours after the test.

Amniocentesis is a generally accepted test, but there are some dangers: the fetus could be injured by the needle, although the baby instinctively moves away from the needle. However, the risks are very slight and the test results are very valuable, particularly for older women.

Among other things, amniocentesis can determine the sex of the fetus and its age, as well as any genetic problems.

BIRTHING DECISIONS

There are several different ways to give birth, each of which enjoys its own followers and advocates. What you decide to do will be partly governed by what your doctor or midwife is willing to do and by what you and your partner decide you want.

The first decision concerns home birth versus hospital or clinic birth. Many people in this country have made this decision a battleground, because they believe that either place is markedly better for baby and mother. Your choice should be determined carefully, in consultation with your medical practitioner and your partner or family members. Generally, doctors do not like home births for the first birth experience. And there are very serious possible complications, when it is absolutely essential that hospital equipment and expertise be immediately available to protect either the baby or you (or both), that rule out a home birth. In order to have a comfortable and safe home birth it is first of all essential that you personally are ideologically committed to the method.

It used to be that hospitals offered only one birthing choice with a long list of "routine procedures." But today, in the face of stiff competition for patients, hospitals have eased up a little and are recognizing the individual patient's needs and desires.

Alternative birthing rooms are a prime example of this aspect of today's hospitals. Designed to offer all the comforts of home with the medical back-up of the hospital, these ABC rooms (as they are usually referred to) are increasingly common in hospitals in major metropolitan areas across the nation. Most are carpeted, decorated like a bedroom with pictures, and sometimes even have a television and small kitchenette. You labor and deliver in the same bed.

Traditional hospitals still use one room for a woman to labor in. It is usually shared; you may not be the only woman laboring there. When delivery is near, the woman is moved onto a wheeled cart (gurney) and transferred to the delivery room. The process of transferring yourself when you are about to deliver, and fighting the urge to push while you are being wheeled down the hall and the doctor suits up, can be very unpleasant. The bright lights and impersonal nature of the delivery room also tend to frighten some women—it seems like you are about to have surgery or that something is very wrong with you, when in fact giving birth is the most natural process in the world.

The Lamaze method, or educated childbirth, is now probably the most common method of giving birth in the U.S. It involves

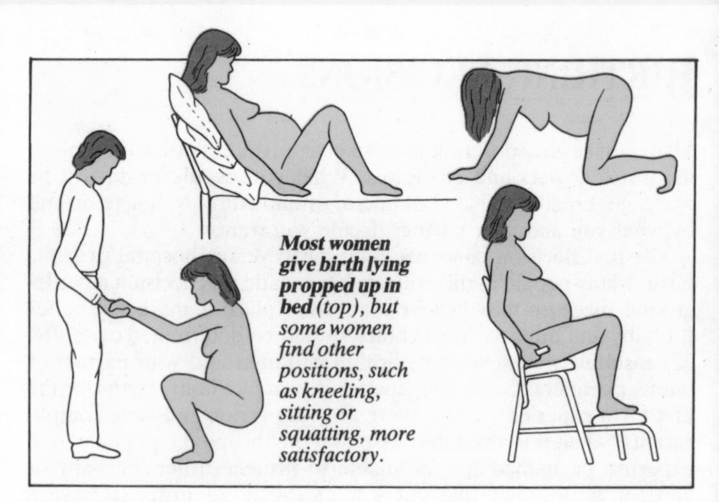

Most women give birth lying propped up in bed *(top), but some women find other positions, such as kneeling, sitting or squatting, more satisfactory.*

minimal medical intervention as the woman labors and delivers with the aid of special breathing and relaxation techniques. These techniques help you control the labor contractions and the pain. Most hospitals require that you take a Lamaze class in the last three months, so that you are familiar with the birth experience and have practiced these techniques.

This method also involves your partner as coach, helping you relax, reminding you of correct breathing, soothing you as you need it, etc. Medication is available as an option, and should be discussed with your doctor or midwife before the birth.

Educated childbirth is often referred to as "natural", but the difficulty is that some women feel pressure to be "organic," that is, go without any medication for pain. Only you (and your doctor and anesthesiologist) can decide about pain medication. Don't let anyone, not your coach or your childbirth teacher or your friends, tell you that you are a failure if you accept medication. This is *your* body and *your* baby.

The Leboyer method centers on the reduction of birth trauma. This trauma, according to Leboyer adherents, is caused by the bright lights, cold steel, and slap on the baby's back by the cold hands of the doctor or midwife. Leboyer says the cry of the newborn is caused by terror and exhaustion brought on by this rough treatment.

The first directive of Leboyer, then, is to dim the lights and warm up the room for the comfort of the naked newborn. Most delivery rooms are kept cool to diminish the possibility of bacteria, and therefore infection. As soon as the baby is born it is placed on the mother's abdomen so bonding and eye-to-eye contact can be made. Noise is kept at a minimum and movements are slow and rhythmic.

Most controversial about Dr. Leboyer is his recommendation that the umbilical cord not be cut immediately but be allowed to cease pulsating, while the baby is lying on its mother's stomach. The newborn is placed in a shallow tub of warm water to approximate the environment it has just left. Sometimes the new father is encouraged to hold his baby gently in the warm water.

There are serious objections to some of the Leboyer recommendations, however, and you should discuss these with your doctor or midwife before you choose this method.

Of course, your choice may be made for you: various complications may dictate that your baby is born by caesarean section. This is considered major surgery, even if you do not have a general anesthetic. Some hospitals allow your partner to be present, but only after viewing a film of what the procedure involves. Some women feel they are "failures" if a caesarean becomes necessary. But remember that the important thing is that a baby is being born. Some women who have experienced both routine delivery and caesarean section say the only difference is when you feel the pain: before the birth with vaginal delivery and after the birth with a caesarean section.

Other choices you will have to make concern pain medication. It is possible, though rare today, to have a general anesthetic (complete unconsciousness), though this is sometimes used in a caesarean. Usually, a general anesthetic is avoided because it is harder for both you and the baby to recover from its effects. A local anesthetic such as an epidural, or saddle block, injected between the vertebrae of the lower back, numbs your body in certain specific areas so that you are awake for the birth, but feeling no pain. However, local anesthesia has serious drawbacks, too, which you should discuss with your doctor or midwife.

Analgesics are any drugs that relieve pain; narcotics, barbiturates, or tranquilizers. You should familiarize yourself with the negatives and positives of these drugs before you go into labor, but don't decide absolutely what you're going to do beforehand: it is important to be open and flexible about painkillers. Many women hold rigidly to the notion that they will not request any pain medication, and have a very hard time in labor as a result. Others ask for pain medication at the slightest twinge. Remember that *all* drugs you take affect your baby, and because its body is so small that effect is more concentrated.

NURSE MIDWIVES

In recent years there have been increasing numbers of certified nurse midwives giving prenatal care and attending births.

Certified nurse midwives (CNM) are nurses who have had additional training and specialize only in routine pregnancy. They attend a normal birth where there is little or no medical intervention needed. They are also trained to recognize when a doctor should be called in—when there is something that is not normal about the birth, such as breech presentation or a prolapsed umbilical cord.

A CNM has had a minimum of six years training, which includes one or more years of practical experience. She follows your pregnancy from the very earliest tests through to after-care, assisting with breast-feeding and other baby needs, as necessary.

Many pregnant women prefer to have a woman attending them, since they believe another woman, who may have gone through the same experience, will be more sympathetic. Since there are very few women obstetrician–gynecologists you are more likely to find a woman CNM.

Other benefits of using a certified nurse midwife are that the cost is usually lower and she will have more time to spend with you and answering your questions. And, when it comes time for labor and delivery, your CNM will usually be close at hand through the whole time.

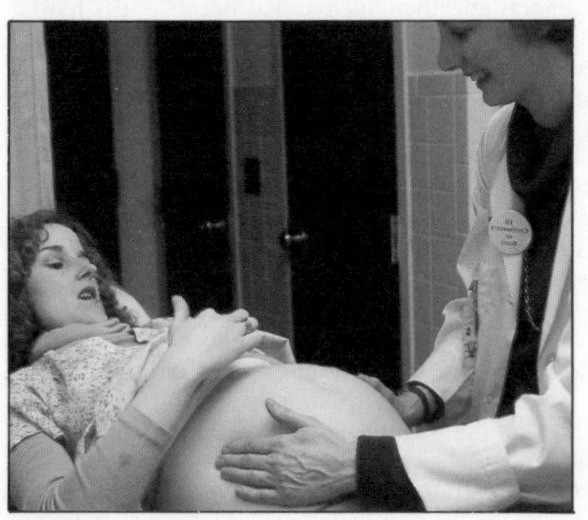

***A nurse midwife** can be a great help, both practically and emotionally, when the time comes for your baby to be born.*

MULTIPLE BIRTHS

It can be exciting but also alarming news to learn that you are carrying more than one fetus and will have twins, or even triplets.

Your genes and the father's genes determine the chances of your conceiving twins (which are the most common form of multiple births). Twins happen in one out of every 85 births.

The discomforts of pregnancy involving twins sometimes feel doubled too. The twins take up more room and thus all the usual troubles with varicose veins, breathlessness, and so on can seem twice as bad than with just a single fetus.

Multiple births are considered a complication of pregnancy for several reasons, and so a doctor (sometimes two) will usually be in attendance at the birth. For example, there is a tendency to go into labor before term when carrying twins, and there are always dangers with premature babies. Unusual presentations of the baby, such as breech (feet- or bottom-first), are also more common with twins.

There are two types of twins: identical and fraternal. With identical twins one egg has been fertilized by one sperm; the babies share one placenta, are the same sex, and will look exactly alike.

With fraternal twins (which are more common), two eggs have been fertilized by two sperm. Fraternal twins have separate placentas. They will not be identical in looks, even if they are the same sex, and will resemble each other just as much as any other brothers and sisters will.

A child's eye color *is determined by the parents' genes. Eyes will be blue only if both genes are blue; if one is brown, this color will be dominant.*

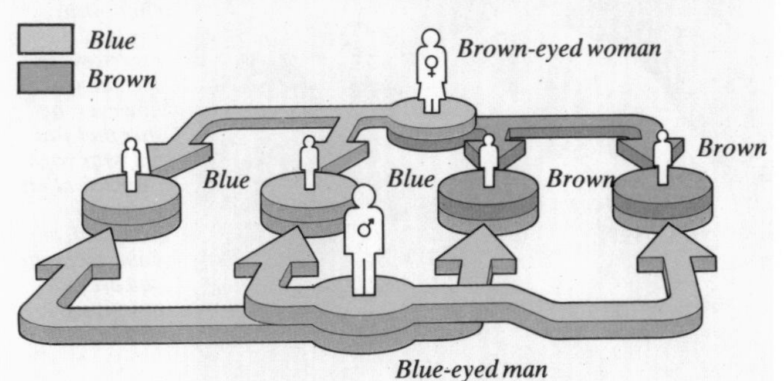

CHILDBIRTH EDUCATION CLASSES

Childbirth education classes are usually required by hospitals if you are going to try for a natural, vaginal delivery, that is, one with a minimum of medication or interference. Even if your doctor or hospital doesn't require classes, it's a good idea to know what to expect in childbirth to help minimize your fear and pain.

Most hospitals and clinics offer childbirth classes, and these are usually less expensive than lessons with a private teacher. You might decide to take lessons with a private teacher, though, if the hospital is not convenient to reach easily every week. All classes are basically the same, with a slight variation in the type of breathing they teach. But the point is always the same: to lessen pain by concentrating on breathing techniques.

Classes usually begin in your seventh month and require that your partner (or a friend) come along as coach. Some men are hesitant about attending classes, at least initially, feeling that it is a woman's job to give birth, and that they don't want any part of it. What they may really be feeling is fear of the birth process. As your partner begins to understand what his job is as your coach, he will probably become more enthusiastic about it. Incidentally, if your partner absolutely refuses to attend your labor and delivery, your childbirth teacher is a good substitute coach.

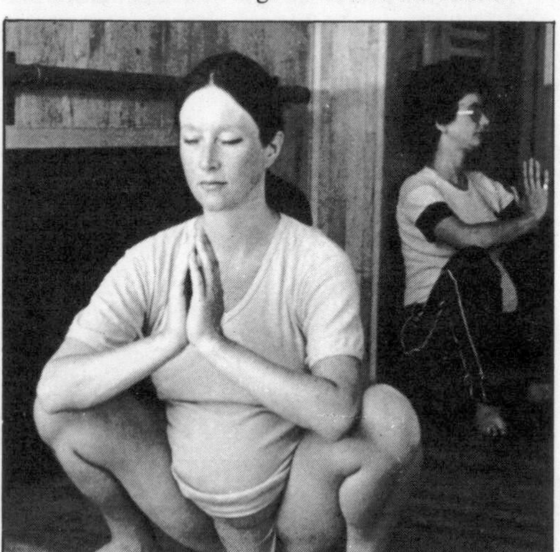

Many women find that special exercises such as yoga *help them enormously in preparing for childbirth. Because these exercises are specialized however, be sure that you tell your yoga instructor that you are pregnant, and your doctor that you are practising yoga.*

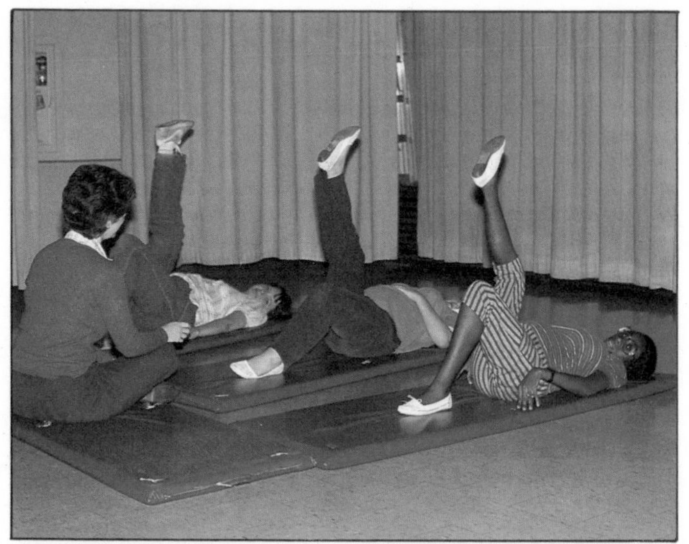

***General exercises** form a key part of many childbirth education classes. They also have advantages beyond the obvious ones of helping you keep in good shape physically. In particular, doing things together with friends and others who are also pregnant is an excellent way of boosting morale, and a valuable way of learning how others are coping and of finding out things that are important to you, but which your doctor might not think to explain.*

Practicing the breathing techniques with your coach is absolutely essential. There is enough going on during labor and delivery that you want to be able to at least do this part of the process semi-automatically.

Classes are also useful for the friendships that are formed with other couples. Many of your friends are probably following the normal pattern and holding off having babies for a few years, so there is a very real need to share information and experiences with others. Childbirth classes are the perfect place to meet other people who are going through the same thing you are, probably for the first time, too. Lifelong friendships have been formed at such classes.

WHAT TO TAKE TO THE HOSPITAL

A few weeks before your due date you should put together a small overnight bag of things you will need while you are in the hospital and things you will need for yourself and the baby to come home again:

- Two pretty nightgowns, front-opening if you intend to breast-feed.
- Bathrobe and slippers.
- Two nursing bras if you intend to nurse, or else a couple of good support bras.
- Several pairs of panties and belts to hold sanitary napkins in place after the delivery. You will have a discharge for several weeks after the birth.
- Personal items: toothbrush, toothpaste, hairbrush, make-up.
- Your "focal point" if you are going to have an educated birth—you will learn about this in childbirth class. This can be anything special or comforting for you—delivery-room nurses have seen plenty of ragged but beloved teddy bears in the arms of grown, laboring women, so don't be embarrassed.
- Clothes for you to leave the hospital in—which will probably be the same ones you wore to the hospital. Your size won't change that much immediately after the birth (so don't get your hopes up too soon).
- Items for the baby: diapers (although the hospital may provide these), tee-shirt, sleeper or coverall, receiving blanket, and a cap.
- Your doctor's telephone number; the hospital and local ambulance or paramedic numbers.
- Items your partner should bring: a camera and film, a list of telephone numbers of relatives and friends, money for the public pay phone, birth announcements.

A dressing gown, panties, nursing bras, skin creams, writing equipment, handi-wipes, soap, sanitary napkins and your "focal point" – a cuddly toy, a shawl or some nightclothes for the baby perhaps – will all be useful for your hospital stay.

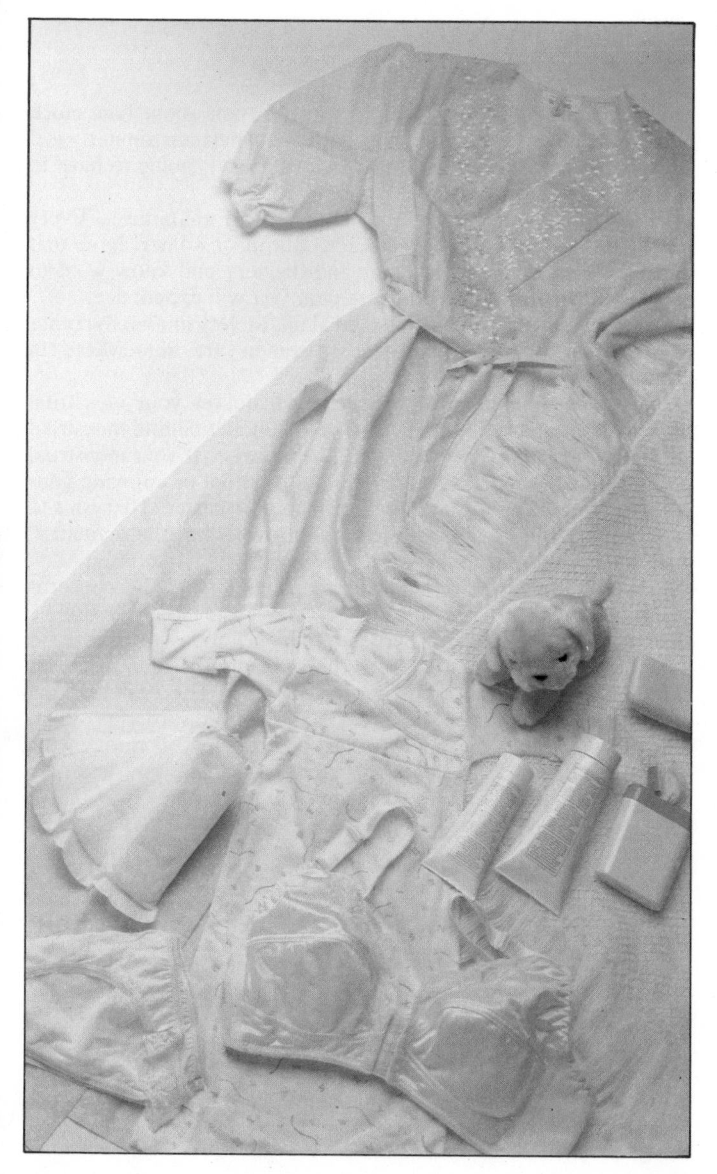

LABOR PAIN

Most women feel a great deal of apprehension about how much labor and delivery is going to hurt (and many partners similarly feel apprehensive about how much their loved one is going to have to endure).

There is no one answer and there are no guarantees. Every individual has a different experience. But most women agree that the more you know about labor and delivery and know what to expect (in general terms), the less pain you will experience.

Some women do not feel any pain at all, or very minimally; other women feel extreme pain. Most women are somewhere in between.

Generally, your labor and delivery will follow your menstrual history. If you have had particularly difficult and painful menstrual cramps, your labor contractions will be likewise. If your menstrual periods never stopped you from going to school or enjoying your regular activities, your labor will probably be easier. That isn't to say that you will be able to carry on enjoying "regular activities" during labor contractions!

Talk to your doctor or midwife about your fears and concerns regarding this issue. They are not "silly" and you will not be "wasting" anyone's time. There is a tendency today to believe we all must be as "natural" as possible and grimly bear whatever comes our way. This is not necessarily true. The best laboring mothers are women who feel as relaxed and in control as possible. And if you need some pain medication to help you through the especially difficult parts of labor, it doesn't make you less of a woman, or a "bad" mother. It means you're human.

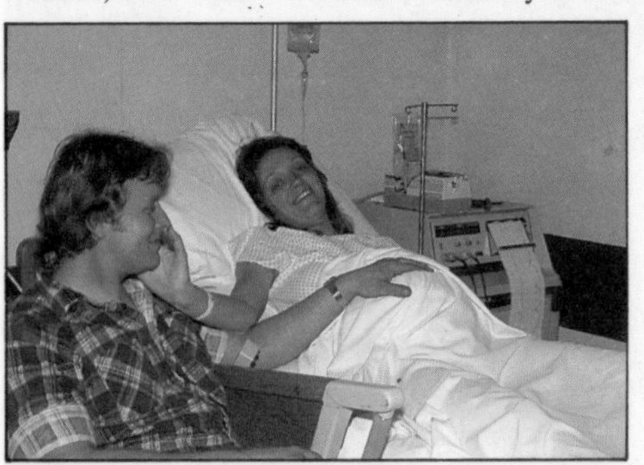

***The experience of labor** is always worrying, and it can be helpful and reassuring to know your partner is nearby.*

STAGES OF LABOR

Engagement, or lightening, usually occurs about two weeks before labor. The baby will settle lower down into your pelvis, usually with its head down. You will know when engagement has occurred because you will be able to breathe easier. This is because the baby will not be exerting so much upward pressure against your ribcage. You will also need to urinate more frequently (if such a thing is possible—you will already think that some days you spend your life urinating).

Most labor begins with a pinkish discharge called the pink or bloody show. The discharge is actually the small mucus plug that has blocked the entrance to the cervix. (Losing the mucus plug does not always mean labor is about to begin; it could still be a few days.) You may be feeling decidedly premenstrual at this point, which is normal since the body function is very similar.

The next thing that happens, if this is really the onset of labor, is that your waters will rupture—your "bag of waters will break." The "water" is the amniotic fluid in which the baby has grown for all these months. There is no warning about when these membranes will break, so be prepared with a sanitary napkin and a plastic sheet on your mattress. The "breaking of the waters" may come as a rush or a trickle, but it does not hurt in any way.

Your uterus may then begin to contract in a rhythmic movement, hardening and relaxing in a kind of wave-like motion. At first the contractions will be no more severe than the cramps of a menstrual period.

Discuss with your doctor in advance when you should go to the hospital. In most cases, you should call your partner, your physician, and the hospital when your water breaks, and be prepared to get to the hospital within a few hours. However, if you have a history of very quick deliveries, or if you have a medical problem, or if your waters have broken earlier than expected, don't delay.

After your waters break, labor and delivery fall into three stages. During the first period, you will have contractions as your cervix widens to allow the baby to pass through it from the womb. This period generally lasts about twelve hours for a first baby and four to eight hours for subsequent babies. However, these are just averages—your labor could be longer or shorter.

By the time your contractions are coming several minutes apart and are fairly intense, you should be at the hospital. Usually by this point you will need the breathing techniques you have been taught

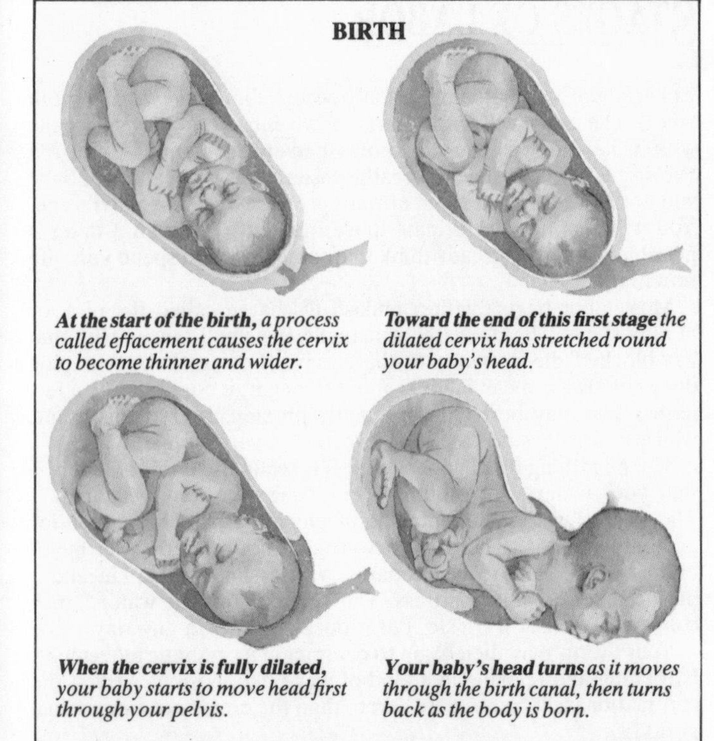

At the start of the birth, *a process called effacement causes the cervix to become thinner and wider.*

Toward the end of this first stage *the dilated cervix has stretched round your baby's head.*

When the cervix is fully dilated, *your baby starts to move head first through your pelvis.*

Your baby's head turns *as it moves through the birth canal, then turns back as the body is born.*

in childbirth class to help you deal with the pain of the contractions. Walk around as much as possible and don't forget to go to the bathroom between contractions.

A transition period occurs when the cervix is fully dilated. Your labor may seem to stop briefly.

Transition is the hardest part of labor. This is when your coach really shines—he should try hard to get you to concentrate and to relax. Now is the time when your cervix dilates to the final size and contractions are very strong and very close together. You really need to concentrate on your breathing techniques now. Don't let anyone interrupt your concentration.

The second stage follows the transition period. Your contractions will become much more powerful and you will feel a strong urge to push the baby down the birth canal. At this point your birth team will help you push only when you are having a contraction. You will find the techniques you learned in childbirth class especially valuable during this period, which often lasts for two to three hours in the case of first children. The second stage ends when the baby emerges from your body and you become a mother!

The second stage is characterized by the overwhelming urge to push, or bear down. Tell the nurses and your coach that you have this urge, but don't push until the doctor or midwife has determined that your cervix is completely open and ready. If you push too soon, you might tear the cervix.

When you are given the green light on pushing and are ready for the delivery room, your coach should put on his sterile clothing as quickly as possible. If he dawdles, he might miss the birth. It also distresses the mother if her coach is gone at this critical time. Pushing is very, very difficult physically, but also very fulfilling. You push during contractions, which usually last about a minute.

When the top of the baby's head is visible it is said to have "crowned." This usually happens after an hour or two of good, strenuous pushing. If it doesn't, the doctor may intervene and use forceps to help the baby come out.

Once the baby is out, the umbilical cord is clamped or cut. Some hospitals invite the father of the child to cut the cord, and surprisingly, despite many misgivings, most fathers do this if given the chance.

The third and final stage of labor is when the placenta (the afterbirth) is pushed out. This usually takes about fifteen to thirty minutes from the time the baby is born. Most women are so excited about the birth and the newborn lying in their arms that they aren't even aware of the placenta's exit. However, since your uterus will continue to contract to expel the placenta, it is possible that you will feel some discomfort. To speed up the process, your doctor may pull gently on the umbilical cord while pressing on your abdomen.

Following the delivery you will probably spend a few hours in a recovery room where a nurse will check your blood pressure and your pulse and massage your uterus to encourage it to begin returning to its normal size. You may want to keep your baby and your partner with you during this time and you should certainly ask if it is possible. Incidentally, if it is not "standard procedure" for this or anything else you want in the way of a birthing experience, you should definitely question the hospital and staff. You have rights, within reason and always with an awareness of the hospital's concern for you and your baby's safety, and these should be honored.

BREAST-FEEDING

The decision to breast-feed is up to you. By your eighth month you should have read everything you can find on the topic, discussed the question with your doctor, asked your partner's opinion, and spoken with other mothers you know who have breast-fed.

Many women worry that breast-feeding will cause their breasts to sag, lose their shape, or even get smaller. Your breasts will definitely get bigger and heavier, and blue veins may appear, but these changes are almost always temporary. If you take care of your breasts during your pregnancy and while you nurse, they will almost certainly return to their original condition when you stop nursing.

If you decide to breast-feed, you should begin preparing your breasts during your eighth month by giving yourself— or asking your partner to give you—a breast massage after taking a shower or bath.

- Support the breast with one hand and massage with the other. You may want to massage in some cocoa butter or a skin lotion.
- Start by placing the fingertips in the underarm area (where the breast glands begin) and gently stroking outward toward the areola (the dark area around the nipple). Next, stroke gently downward from the collar bone.
- Gently massage the nipple between the thumb and first and second fingers. It will harden and expand—the bigger and firmer your nipples, the easier it will be for the baby to suck from them.
- Repeat for the other breast.

Believe it or not, breast-feeding is not necessarily an easy or automatic thing. There are many problems that may arise, and you should be prepared for the possibility that you may not be able to breast-feed for some reason or other. But usually patience and dedication will win the day. There are doctors who specialize in nursing problems. And the nurses at the hospital will help you, as will the pediatrician and midwife who attended your prenatal care and delivery.

After your delivery, it usually takes about two to three days for your milk to "come in." Until then, a yellowish, sticky fluid called colostrum is secreted. Your new baby will suck this because it contains needed proteins and antibodies—it's perfectly normal.

There are two basic things that must happen to breast-feed successfully: the baby must learn to suck and your body must learn to give up its milk to the baby.

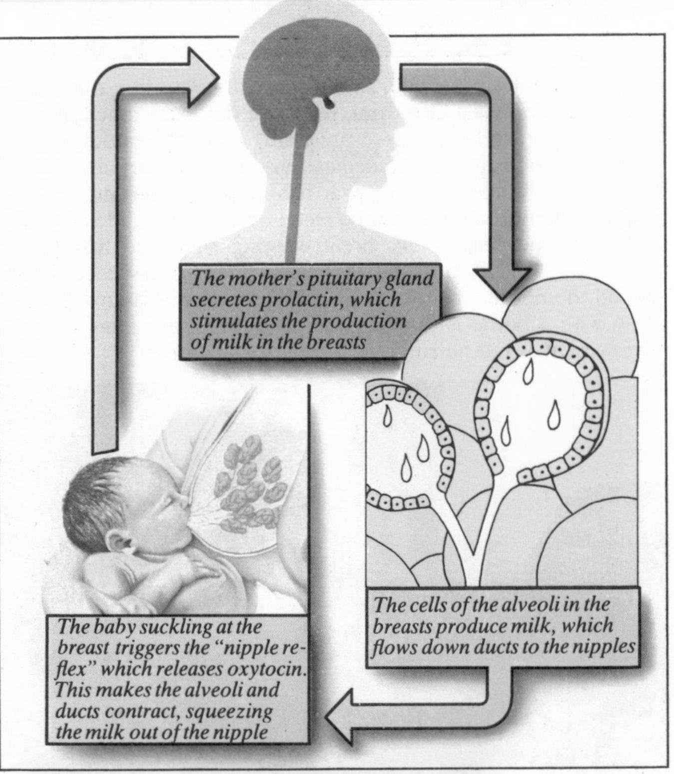

The mother's pituitary gland secretes prolactin, which stimulates the production of milk in the breasts
The cells of the alveoli in the breasts produce milk, which flows down ducts to the nipples
The baby suckling at the breast triggers the "nipple reflex" which releases oxytocin. This makes the alveoli and ducts contract, squeezing the milk out of the nipple

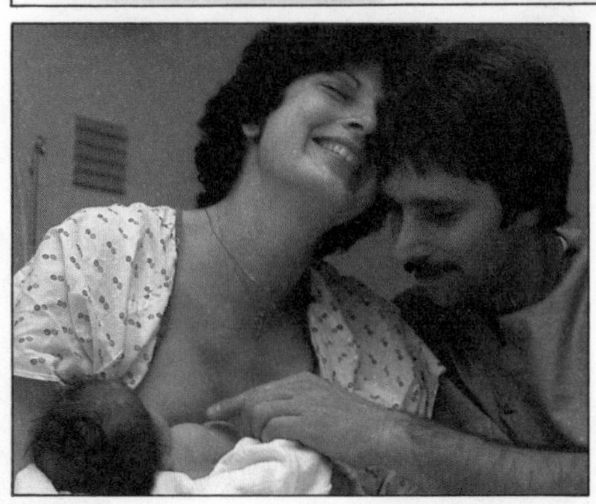

Your breasts contain ducts *that connect the thousands of tiny, milk-secreting alveoli to the nipple like the tributaries of a river. During pregnancy hormones from the placenta cause the breasts to enlarge and prepare them for producing milk.*

It is important for your milk supply that you stay calm and relaxed. You must also drink plenty of fluids (as much, if not more, than while you were pregnant) and eat healthily. You should also avoid certain medications, and even certain foods, which can be passed on to your baby through your milk.

Be patient if all does not go well immediately (and very few mothers and babies get breast-feeding right the first time around). And if you find that you cannot breast-feed your child, do not feel guilty or think of yourself as a failure. Feeding with a bottle is just as good. The important thing is that your baby is fed nutritiously so that it can thrive.

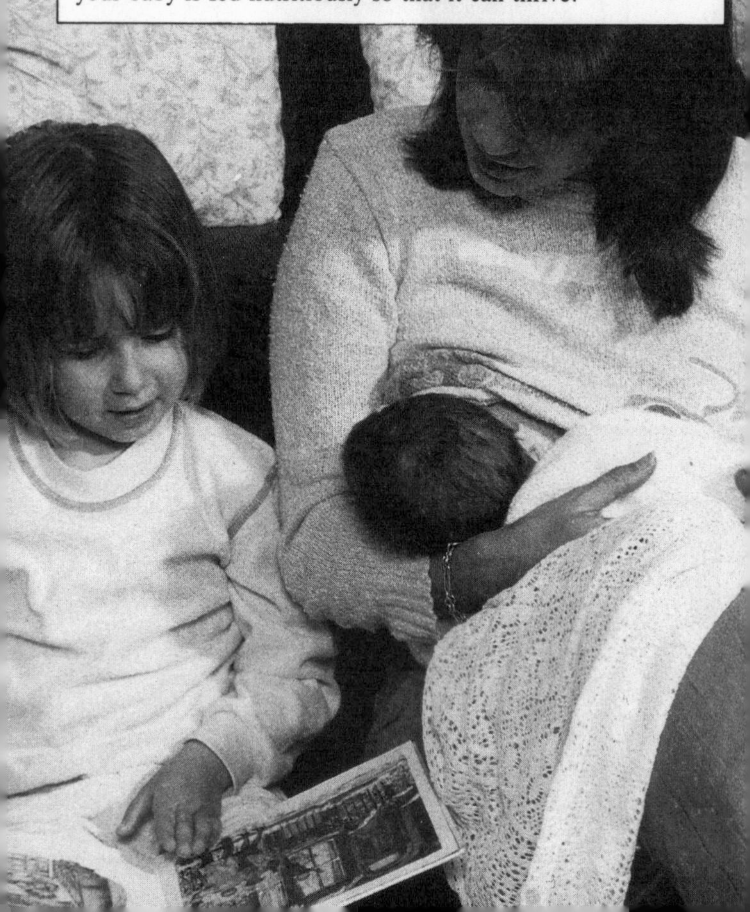

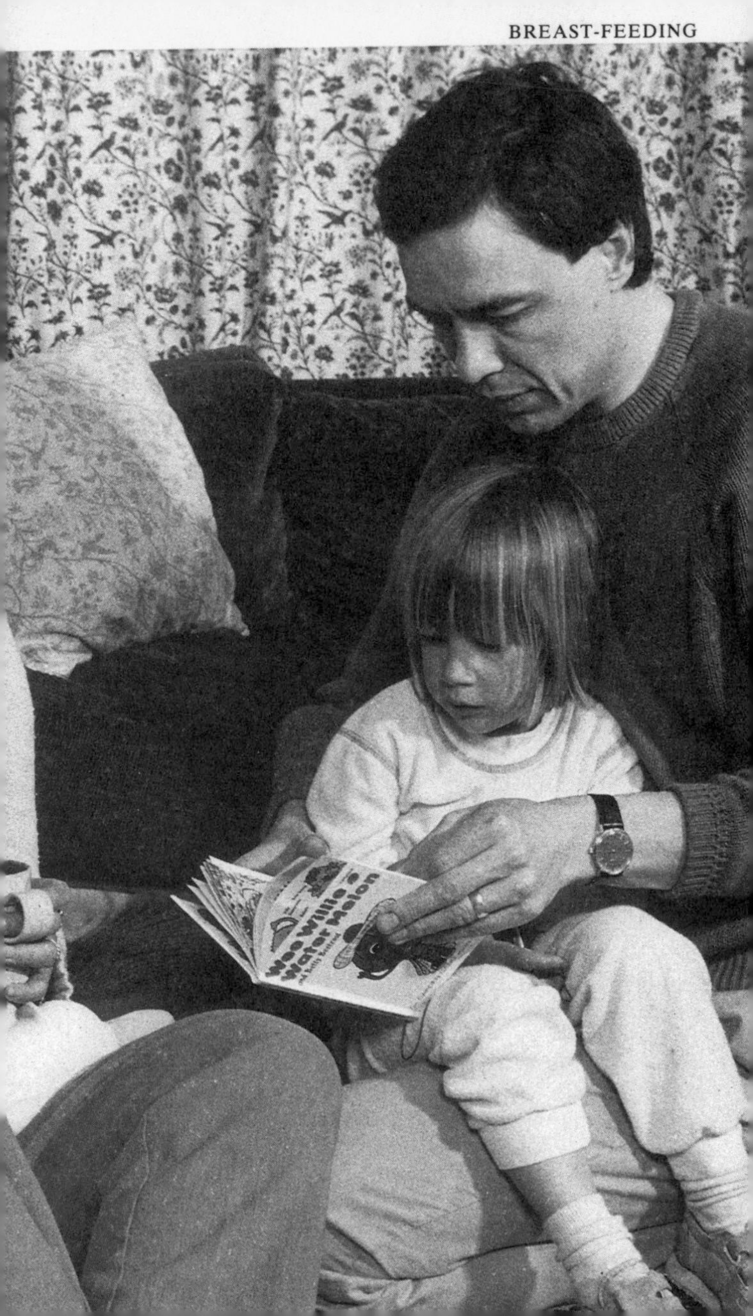
Wee Willie
Water Melon

GLOSSARY

AFTERBIRTH. *See* Placenta.
AMNIOCENTESIS. A test of the amniotic fluid surrounding the baby to determine whether there are any chromosomal defects.
AREOLA. The colored area around the nipple.
BREECH BIRTH. A birth where the baby is born feet or buttocks first, instead of head first.
CAESAREAN SECTION. The delivery of the baby by making a surgical incision into the uterus.
CERVIX. The lower end of the uterus; it is constricted and projects into the vagina.
CHLOASMA. Also called "mask of pregnancy." Brown spots on the face and upper body.
COLOSTRUM. A yellowish, sticky fluid containing proteins and antibodies, secreted by the breasts during pregnancy and for the first few days after birth.
ECLAMPSIA. A rare complication of pregnancy, characterized by sudden high blood pressure and protein in the urine.
EDEMA. Excess fluid retention, which may cause swelling.
EMBRYO. An unborn baby from conception through to the third month.
EPISIOTOMY. An incision made during delivery between the vagina and the anus to avoid tearing the mother's tissues.
FETAL MONITOR. Any device used to measure the heart rate of the fetus.
FETUS. An unborn baby from the third month onward.
GERMAN MEASLES (RUBELLA). A mild childhood illness that can cause serious birth defects if a pregnant woman contracts it.
GESTATION. The nine-month period from conception to delivery.
HEMORRHOIDS. Swollen blood vessels that become painful swellings in the anus.
INCONTINENCE. Inability to control the flow of urine.
KEGEL EXERCISES. Exercises designed to strengthen the pelvic floor.
LABOR. The process during which the baby leaves the womb and passes through the birth canal.
NATURAL CHILDBIRTH. Also called "prepared" or "educated" childbirth. Giving birth with aid of breathing and relaxation techniques to reduce or eliminate the need for drugs.
OB-GYN. Short for obstetrician-gynecologist; that is, a doctor specializing in pregnancy and female reproductive problems.

Placenta. The organ that forms on the lining of the womb during pregnancy and provides the baby with nourishment and oxygen through the umbilical cord. It also carries away the baby's waste products. Also called the "afterbirth," since it is expelled from the body after delivery.

Placenta previa. A condition where the placenta lies between the baby and the birth canal.

Postpartum. The period after the birth of a child.

Postpartum depression. Feelings of sadness or depression following the birth of a baby.

Pre-eclampsia. A disorder of late pregnancy where the mother's blood pressure rises sharply and she retains fluid.

Spider veins. Also called "spider angiomas" or "spider nevae." Spidery red marks that may appear on the face, neck or shoulders.

Stretch marks. Also called "striae." Reddish streaks that can occur on the abdomen, breasts, hips, and buttocks, caused by hormonal changes and stress on the skin.

Toxemia. *See* Eclampsia.

Trimester. One of the three three-month periods into which pregnancy is divided.

Umbilical cord. The cord that connects the placenta to the fetus.

Urethra. The canal that carries urine off from the bladder.

Varicose vein. An enlarged or swollen vein in the leg.

INDEX

Page numbers in *italic* refer to the illustrations and captions

Credits:

Art Director: Peter Bridgewater
Editorial Consultants: Maria Pal/Clark Robinson Ltd

Picture credits:

The author and publishers have made every effort to identify the copyright owners of the photographs; they apologize for any omissions and wish to thank the following:

Creszentia Allen, 56; Artemis/Hartigan, 25, 34, 69, 78, 89b; Jessica Beard, 90–91; Paul Forrester, 54, 83; John Heseltine, 45; Ian Howes, 46; Lifecircle, 63, 68, 81, 84; Mothers Work, 41, 49; Chris Thomson, 39.